TRUE TALES OF
ORGANISATIONAL LIFE

career, great choice of career!

Barbara
X.

TRUE TALES OF ORGANISATIONAL LIFE

Barbara-Anne Wren

KARNAC

First published in 2016 by
Karnac Books Ltd
118 Finchley Road
London NW3 5HT

British Library Cataloguing in Publication Data

A C.I.P. for this book is available from the British Library

ISBN-13: 978-1-78220-189-2

Typeset by Medlar Publishing Solutions Pvt Ltd, India

Printed in Great Britain

www.karnacbooks.com

For
Matt and Mary
Jim and Peg
Josephine and Tom

And in loving memory
of my Dad
and of Connell

Thank you for getting the stories started

... what really gets us is the undertow: what is not being said.
The not-said is so ferociously important.

Ali Smith, The Guardian, *June 6, 2015*

CONTENTS

ACKNOWLEDGEMENTS

There are so many people who sustained me in the work described here, and the writing of this book. I would like to thank them. The late Riva Miller who was my wise and kind mentor when I first started working at the Royal Free. Halina Brunning for constant and invaluable support, throughout all these years. My psychology family, the occupational health psychology network: Clare Allen, Anthony Schwartz, Teresa Jennings, Jan Hill-Tout, Leslie Morrison, and Paul Flaxman for support, community, creativity, and fun, as we all developed our psychology services. My psychology friends: Britt Tajet-Foxall for listening to so many stories, and helping me to keep thinking about crafting and positioning. Anthony Schwartz for always supporting me in my writing. Chris D'Netto for kind, sensitive support and encouragement especially in the final stages of writing the book. To my writing group, Caroline Greene and Nora Hughes, thank you for writing support through the years, especially Caroline for the final edit, and thanks also to David Mullany for help with editing the seven tales. Thank you to Glenda Fredman for her inspirational work embedding systemic ideas in psychology services, and for many helpful conversations and training days, and Lih-Mei Liao for wise supervision, and still thinking space.

Thank you to all the clinicians and managers who allowed their stories to be told, to all the clients of the psychology service from whom I learnt so much, and to all my Royal Free colleagues, who have given me support, encouragement, the chance to be creative and who have been so supportive of this book. Thanks especially to Dr Adrian Tookman who invited me to be the Schwartz Round facilitator and to my co-facilitator Dr Mark Harber. Thank you to all the participants of the Royal Free Rounds for their enthusiasm, honesty, insights, and generous sharing of experience. Thank you very much also to the original team who brought Schwartz Rounds to the UK: Jocelyn Cornwell and Joanna Goodrich at The Point of Care Foundation now and originally at the Kings Fund, and Leslie Morrison and Sean Elyan at Gloucester Hospitals NHS Foundation Trust, and to everyone at The Point of Care Foundation. Thank you to Marjorie Stanzler and Beth Lown at The Schwartz Center for Compassionate Healthcare in Boston and everyone there for their warm welcomes when we visited. Special thanks to the first wave of UK Schwartz Round facilitators and medical leads: Raymond Chadwick, Jenny Watmore-Eve, Anne Cullen, Andrew Knight, Jennifer Todd, John Pepper and Geraldine McVeigh for the very enjoyable opportunity to work with you all and to develop new thinking about implementing Schwartz Rounds in the UK. And to my family and friends for all their love and support, thank you all so much.

ABOUT THE AUTHOR

Barbara-Anne Wren is a chartered psychologist and organisational consultant working privately and in the NHS. In 1999 she set up the in—house psychology service for staff at Royal Free London Foundation Trust providing therapy, coaching, mediation, facilitation, team and organisational development interventions. Later she led on the successful piloting of Schwartz Rounds at the Royal Free, one of the two national UK Schwartz Round pilot sites. As lead psychologist at the Point of Care Foundation, she then led on the development and implementation of of the national training and mentoring programme for Schwartz Round clinical leads and facilitators. As chair and founder member of the UK National Network of Practitioner Occupational Health Psychologists, she has worked nationally and internationally to develop theory and practice to improve staff experience in healthcare settings. She is a consultant psychologist and Schwartz Round lead at Royal Free London NHS Foundation Trust, director of Wren Psychology Associates, and a visiting lecturer at City University, London. She is an associate fellow, and a member of the Health, Occupational and Coaching Divisions of the British Psychological Society, and a member of OPUS.

INTRODUCTION

In 1999 a London teaching hospital decided to establish an innovative psychology post. The post would be dedicated to staff and would be split in two, half of the time providing individual therapeutic services to staff members, and the remaining time working at an organisational level. It would be based in a well established and highly regarded occupational health unit where there had been a part-time psychology presence until then, and there was a multidisciplinary team of doctors and nurses. The unit had recently published a review of staff health—or rather ill health (Williams, Michie, & Pattani, 1998)—in the NHS, making the case for investment in the health of NHS staff to promote well-being, effectiveness, and productivity, which had helped to secure funding for this post. The post offered a tremendous opportunity and an overwhelming task. There were 5000 staff in the hospital at the time, high rates of stress and disillusionment throughout the NHS, and there was no clear blueprint for a post like this—though at the time coincidentally (or not) there were a number of psychologists being appointed to similar posts in the UK.[1] Added to this challenge was the widely held

---

[1]This coincidence led to the establishment of the national network of occupational health practitioner psychologists.

perception of psychology as a resource that offered individual solutions to distressed staff. The hope was maybe that they could disappear through the portal of occupational health to emerge fully intact and ready to work hard, after an invisible and mysterious intervention that had taken away stress, banished emotion, and smoothed the edges of personalities that fitted uncomfortably with, or snagged against, their respective colleagues, teams, and work tasks. This perception located the problem, and by implication the solution, within the individual staff member.

The aim of this book is to describe the work that was developed in response to this challenge which, rather than banishing emotion and distress, was concerned to manage meaning and complexity, understand emotional life at both an organisational and individual level, and create spaces in which the unique challenges of healthcare work could be observed and understood. The importance of context, of careful listening, and of storytelling at all organisational levels will be described, along with the crucial role of systemic and narrative approaches in the work. Throughout the book reflections will be made on developing the role of psychology, and how positioning and flexibility enhanced and expanded this role. The use of metaphor and the consideration of interventions at their symbolic level as well as in terms of their content will be discussed. The vital role of creativity in sustaining staff and managing hope will be highlighted and links made to other creative endeavours: storytelling and performance, all of which sophisticated activities achieve an outcome that could be described simply as the settling impact of telling *and* hearing stories that resonate and validate, create community, and reduce isolation.

The book is divided into the following sections. Part I describes the evolution of the role of psychology in a large teaching hospital with a particular focus on how the service was developed to be responsive to context, and used relevant theory to frame its responses to staff in difficulty. Four case studies or "tales" are described. They illuminate the themes considered and were pivotal in further developing the service. Part II begins with an overview of NHS culture and then describes how a new intervention, Schwartz Rounds, was brought to the UK from America and positioned to be responsive to this culture. The way in which the process of implementation was shaped to ensure that the space it created could allow for a consideration of layers of context and meaning, both local and national will be described. In Part III the specific process of implementing this intervention in the teaching hospital will be described with reference to the work outlined in Part I, and also to the subtle process of crafting private stories for a public telling using systemic theory and psychological understanding. Part IV includes seven stories told at Rounds, each one illustrating a core aspect of staff experience of healthcare work. Part V is a closing reflection on the experience of working in healthcare and the emotional challenges it poses.

The book moves from the general to the specific, and from the professional to the personal in each section. It aims to continually consider the interaction between context and emerging interventions and to suggest ways to conceptualise these interventions drawing on a range of psychological theories and skills. All of the work described was done at the same hospital by the author with the exception of some of Part II, which includes reflections on work undertaken within a national level role the author had at the time. All details of stories have been altered to protect confidentiality, and all the clinicians and other healthcare staff whose stories are included have provided consent. On occasions and particularly towards the end of the book, the author becomes the "I" of a story or experience, as the impact of the work is described through the impact it had on her. The storytelling becomes more personal as the book progresses and moves towards the specific, and the individual experience. The views and ideas expressed are the author's alone and the book aims to trace an emerging understanding of the multi-layered nature of healthcare work and of how best to creatively and responsively implement interventions with reference to the experiences of a psychologist working as both therapist and an internal consultant.

PART I

Levels of context, layers of meaning

*Evolving a role for psychology
in a London hospital*

What are stories for?

They give a shape to experience, they form us as we speak them, carve us as we write them. They connect our body to our mind, our inner to our outer world, our mind to our heart, our muscle to our bones, and link movement to stillness.

A role for psychology in organisational life:
linking movement and stillness

Wheels within wheels: the context of healthcare is relationship

The treatment that patients receive in healthcare settings is delivered through a relationship: a relationship with a caregiver, a medical team, a nursing and therapy team, a healthcare organisation and, in the UK, with a national system that has both symbolic and actual power and meaning. Elements at different levels of this relationship will influence the experience and the outcomes for patients. And at the heart of healthcare are many, many individual interactions. The ways in which they take place have the opportunity to cure, heal, soothe, comfort, educate, generate hope and a feeling of safety, and enable and give control to patients. Of course they also have the potential for the opposite of each of these effects: to create fear, anxiety, and anger, misunderstanding, a sense of helplessness and hopelessness, and a resistance to treatment.

Depending on their own resources, knowledge, and motivation, and the design of their role and work, healthcare staff will have different levels of ability to provide these vital elements of the patient experience, and different skills and insight into their impact on their patients and the emotional experience of patients (and colleagues). They may also differ in the training they have had, their access to and use of support, and their understanding of how support may help them in their development. Another key difference may be in the extent to which they are contained and kept safe by the management systems and structures (including teams) in which they are working. That is, the extent to which they are free from undue worry and provided with enough clarity and support to work efficiently. And whether they have enough space to process work experiences, in order to work effectively and to use interdependencies productively. They may also vary in the amount of time available to them to attend to the non-technical aspects of their work, and in their confidence to manage the relationship with their patient as an instrument for healing and compassion. They may have more or less insight into the extent to which this relationship can dramatically improve the patient experience, even at a time of bad news and bleak prognoses.

Within this broad-brush picture there are of course many variations. Different specialties make different demands. Some are more physically demanding, others more emotionally challenging. Some are both. Others are very technical. In many areas of healthcare work now, staff are integrating sophisticated technology into the provision of care. Some patients are very ill, others have simple, treatable illnesses, and others have long-term chronic conditions. Some people are in hospital to have their babies, a time of optimism and hope, others to have their final illness. And some come in with a simple illness and things deteriorate unexpectedly. Some are planned admissions, others unplanned, with all the background trauma that implies.

Organisational life in healthcare: keeping the wheels turning

And within a hospital, as well as doctors, nurses and therapists, so many other staff work behind the scenes. There are managers whose role is to link strategic understanding and operational reality and who need to have a conceptual overview to ensure that the day to day routine runs effectively. They must ensure that their staff are skilled enough, strong enough, well enough, connected to each other enough, to do their daily work. They are increasingly torn between a focus on the working of their staff and a pull towards the management of the challenges and competition from the outside world, the challenges that need to be attended to, in order to secure the future of the work and the organisation. Many fall between the gaps in this dichotomy.

There are porters who see everything that happens as they bring worried patients to and from procedures, tests, and operations that can decide the outcome of their illness and the shape of their future lives. There are cleaners who contribute to the everyday human contact that keeps patients in touch with the world outside, and make them feel like a person not a patient. There are laboratory staff who analyse results and see a story emerging through the way cells are dividing or blood is clotting. Sometimes they know the patient's fate even before the doctor does. There are scientists who plan treatments to give a patient the best chance, the most hopeful way forward. And so many more staff, all of them absorbing an ever-increasing volume of work at a time of massive uncertainty about the future and the shape of healthcare delivery. Every single day a huge number of people are in constant motion in a hospital ensuring that it is run effectively and that patients feel cared for and are seen, diagnosed, and treated effectively and appropriately, and as quickly as possible.

Regardless of the reason they are in hospital, all patients have crossed the boundary between sickness and health. All have families who want them back on the other side. The patient and his family need the health-care system and all the staff whose energy keeps it turning, to give them safe passage back to health and hope. For some this will be possible and for others it will not. This is the burden that healthcare staff carry as they go about their busy day. It is within the interactions that take place during each day that hope meets reality, and healthcare staff must facilitate the transformation that ensues, for a patient and his family: the delicate adjustments of expectation and of understanding; the appreciation of the meaning of what life will be like from now on.

To achieve this clinicians must draw together the expertise of their colleagues and all of their own understanding of the patient's condition and prognosis, to provide information and treatment with sensitivity, wise use of the emotional context, and an appreciation of the patient's ability to understand, absorb, receive, and adjust. They must balance certainty and uncertainty in deciding what position to take in relation to the information and treatment they will provide, while making sure they don't miss anything important in their diagnosis. They need to use their creativity to blend the art with the science of medicine and incorporate their understanding of the subtle influence of time on adjustment to illness and disability into their pacing of the delivery of information. While staying mindful of the importance of pacing they know that organisations are giving them less and less time in which to work. And finally they must try to enable a patient to manage his dependence on the healthcare system in a way that allows him to achieve the optimum balance between retaining and relinquishing control, in order to protect his physical and mental health going forward. This complex, emotionally significant work takes place in minutes, over and over again throughout the day. Once it is finished, the clinician always knows that the next patient is waiting and that for the patient this is the only appointment of the day.

The large cogs of the hospital wheel keep moving and contain within them thousands of these vital and meaningful turns. Each small turn contains a consultation in which the clinician's ability to be sensitive to the multiple layers of context profoundly impacts on a patient and his family's ability to understand the present, and to accept and digest the shape of the future.

Something catches, the wheel stops turning, a memory comes to mind

Sometimes the wheel turns smoothly and sometimes something jars. Maybe the clinician is too tired, not supported, or not clear. Lately the opportunities for creativity and using the art of medicine are being challenged by the introduction of pathways and protocols, the reduction of skill to a set of competencies, a series of "simple" steps. Clinicians can feel restricted and limited. Anxiety[2] develops about deviating from protocols, when clinical intuition suggests other routes. Or maybe the work is poorly designed, the roles and teams too loosely structured. Perhaps a team have lost their way. Or the patient or the family refuse to accept reality. Or the sheer volume of the work is too much to bear. Perhaps the organisation is not coherent enough and the ambiguity leads to conflict between staff. Or a group of managers lose authority for some reason and staff lose containment and clarity. A mutinous culture develops. Perhaps a terrible death happens on a ward and traumatises staff. Or a member of staff has a mental health problem, which affects colleagues' ability to keep the wheels turning. Sometimes an error is made and the clinician loses confidence. Or one part of the organisation moves out of sync with another and clinicians grow angry as they feel their work is being delayed in ways they cannot influence. Or the organisation's priorities change and a clinician is wrong-footed. Maybe a piece of work is too close to home or simply too sad, and a team cannot come to terms with it. Committed, engaged staff are seen to grow tired and burn out. Two members of a team refuse to speak and the team is unable to function.

Suddenly the psychologist comes to mind.

---

[2]Anxiety both conscious and unconscious will be referred to throughout this book in relation to the experience of work. It can be simply defined as "what threatens to swamp the capacity for understanding, thinking, and the sense of self" (see Armstrong & Rustin, 2015, for this definition and a detailed discussion of the concept). Their recent book was written in part as a reassessment of the concept of anxiety at work originally described in a classic paper by Menzies (1960). See also Menzies Lyth (1988).

Ruptures and hidden possibilities

Over and over again at times of rupture, fear, uncertainty, loss, conflict, inability to mobilise, energise, and move forward, difficulties in digesting, or understanding an experience, the psychologist would come to mind. A request would come in, an invitation to do some work. "Can you help?" the organisation would ask. "X has happened and we thought of you." The invitations would arrive laden with many different meanings and assumptions: about the nature of problems, and the rules of organisational life; about the possibilities of solutions and who could generate them; about what aspects of experience the organisation wanted to own and disown, as the many wheels kept turning. Each response positioned the psychology work in relation to the organisation, with reference to the best use of limited resources and the most constructive next step for the individual and the organisation. The development of each intervention contributed to an emerging understanding of how the service could shape itself to be responsive, while remaining sensitive to the reality of individual experience and the pressures of organisational imperatives.

Positioning psychology: ambivalence, vulnerability, and strength

What does it mean to be a psychologist in a busy organisation? Where would you place yourself? What does it mean to have your own psychologist working in your hectic hospital? How would you use her?

Everyone is fascinated by psychology, drawn towards it, and a little bit uncertain about it. Everyone wants to be a psychologist, or is one, or knows one. They are a bit afraid too. People worry that psychologists can read their minds, see things they like to keep hidden, know things that are unknowable. If only. They worry that their vision is maybe four-dimensional, when theirs is just three-dimensional. They ask questions at parties that boil down to questions about what psychologists can see, what they know, and how can they know it. They need to believe that it can do something and they project fear and hope into it, mostly about whether it can be potent.

When they are in crisis they rely blindly on the potency they give it. Immobilised by the force of their own emotional experience they pray it will unravel the correct thread that will enable them to take shape coherently again. When they feel strong, they often dismiss it. For it is so complicated finding the right way to acknowledge complexity. The right words to convey the fact that we all live in parallel universes within which happiness and sadness can share a single moment, strength can emerge from huge trauma or dissipate completely, life can seem just fine on the outside while extreme difficulty or illness are being managed behind the scenes on a minute by minute basis, and everything can change in a heartbeat.

They suspect that psychologists are not fully one of them and that it is the psychologist's own vulnerability and history that has drawn her to this work in the first place. They are glad to leave the vulnerability identity with the psychologist. But where should they put her? They are unsure of her place in the hustle and bustle of the marketplace that is modern working life. Psychologists can be unsure too. There are so many cracks they could fall through, so many ways in which the ambivalence might trip them up. It is hard to know how to integrate it all, the mystery, the banality, the humdrum, the ugly, the difficult, and the beautiful. Though there is something hopeful about a profession that does try to integrate it, that aims to create something productive and meaningful from chaos and confusion, not by imposing truths but by allowing form to emerge. By crafting wisely so that it can be productively seen. But it is not an easy task.

For in this busy, busy, modern competitive world of work that we have created, we are unsure how much time we have to pay attention to complexity or to beauty or transience, or problems with no easy solution, how much permission we have to say where we actually are, rather than where we think we should be. We are preoccupied by where we need to be to win the games of organisational life. The need to succeed can narrow our lens and make us blind to the meaning of the problems we encounter.

Organisational life: the difficulty and importance of thinking systemically

"Things fall apart the centre cannot hold" (Yeats, 1919)

We are ambivalent about meaning at so many levels. At a societal level we now carry a fear of a "catastrophic loss of meaning" (Armstrong & Rustin, op. cit.) as the problems we face become so complex. The conceptual understanding, the emotional energy needed to truly appreciate and address organisational complexity is so potentially overwhelming. We worry that we cannot carry this burden; we do not have the resources. The resources needed are emotional and intellectual resources: the ability to be creative and consistent, and to persevere despite great risks and uncertainty, though this reality often becomes lost in translation and then obscured by a focus on financial resources. We seem to have an unconscious default, within which we keep reducing the mysterious to the mundane, complexity to a quick fix, the unsolvable to a single solution. In this way we stay partially blind and unable to gather up the courage, energy, and vision we know we now need to have to respond creatively at a time of huge challenge and uncertainty in individual and organisational life. Also we like power, and we like to win. We need the tools to win. Even if the battle is with ourselves.

So we fall in love with one-dimensional interventions. Under time pressure we want to find the *one* solution that will solve our problems, keep us sane, make life manageable, and make organisations viable. Thoughtful, slowed down, integrated interventions feel too expensive and time-consuming, emotional life too diffuse and unknowable (though never has our theoretical understanding of emotional development been more promising and exciting), organisational life feels precarious, uncontaining, and disappointing. Rational approaches to our problems carry the comfort of concreteness and certainty. Though at the same time we continue to love stories and narrative and the way in which they still surprise us even though we know that all the stories must be told by now. We like the jolt and the shift they produce, the alchemy of the expected with the unexpected, the containment with the challenge (see Bruno Bettelheim, 1976).

It is an interesting time for psychology. It has so much of importance to offer, but people are so ambivalent about it. It is sometimes ambivalent about itself. Could it all be reduced to a simple manual? What is the cheapest way to provide it? How can we prove it works? Can its essence be reduced to a commodity?

But the essence of psychology is in relationship. It is dynamic, not a static piece of content. It works because it moves. For it is in the bringing of theory, skill, and conceptual understanding into a relationship—a relationship with many layers—that the power of psychology emerges. At its best it engages quickly, responds carefully, considers slowly, steps wisely, and knows how to position itself to create shape and meaning.

It is elusive and potent and its work develops delicately from the orchestration of the interplay of elements.

It uses story to organise the elements, emotion to understand them, and intellect and theory to decide how best to take the next steps, what way to put one foot in front of the other in order to create meaning. It aims to help individuals and organisations to do this too. And it works with them on digesting the emotional impact of the relationship between the person and his experience, in order to correctly connect all the relevant elements for understanding to emerge. It facilitates moments of stillness in order to create space for this process to occur. In this way it moves in the opposite direction to organisational life. It pushes against the busyness to make space for individuals and teams, to think, to be creative, and to feel enough; space to ensure they can remain realistically responsive to the reality of their life and their work, their relationship with their organisation, their colleagues, and patients, and ultimately with themselves, in order to make wise moves forward.

This is the story of the creation of space, and the emergence of a psychology role in one organisation—a large teaching hospital in London at the beginning of this century, the story of the development of one relationship between the context of healthcare and the context of psychology.

Stress, distress, and hidden meaning: accessing therapy at work

The most obvious association to the idea of a psychologist is that of a therapist. It is in the realm of therapy that the uses of psychology are best known and in the early days of the psychology service this was the way in which the organisation and its staff were keen to position the role. Referrals came through quickly and were very varied: a nurse who was suddenly suffering from panic attacks when moving from a ward to a clinic based job and unable to understand why; an Asian man nearing retirement feeling bullied and overtaken by his much younger white manager; a recently promoted young woman finding it very difficult to manage staff who had previously been friends, and an oncologist feeling weary and exhausted by the more cost-conscious context within which cancer care is being delivered. Many of these individuals were experiencing high levels of distress that they mostly tried to keep hidden and were very fearful of being unable to continue to work. They were also worried about what the feeling of distress and the fear of being overwhelmed would mean for their family roles and ultimately for their view of themselves. Many hoped to keep the problem hidden at work.

A psychologist in an organisation is instantly associated with "stress" and staff consider that use of the psychology service will be an antidote. So they use the service in a number of different ways and for a variety of reasons but they all share this hope of the antidote, or a removal of pain and banishment of distress. They wonder:

How can you help me manage the fear that without structure and support I will be revealed for the fake that I am?

How can you return me to normal so I can resume my job without choking on the humiliation and shame I am being made to feel?

How can you help me persuade myself that it is silly to worry about what my friends think of me and to be frightened about the possibility of losing them and feeling very alone in my decision–making?

How can you stop me feeling the anguish of worrying about providing inadequate care?

Responding to requests for intervention required sensitivity not only to conscious and unconscious hopes but also to a consideration of the meaning and the context of referrals. The work aimed to introduce this meaning into the therapeutic work, and also to feed this meaning back into the organisation.

Bringing messages from the organisation

Individuals accessing therapy[3] bring with them stories, stories about the past and tentative stories of the future. In the foreground, however, are stories of the present. These stories in particular are presented as needing readjustment, transformation, and sometimes the hope of a removal of, or recasting, of some of the key players, including occasionally the clients themselves. In relation to work problems clients most often hope to recast or remove the character of their manager or a significant colleague in the drama that has taken hold of them.

---

[3]*Therapy* will be used to refer to individual therapeutic work, *psychology* to the overall psychology service.

While the movement of therapy is from a focus on the external stage of the work context to reconsideration and recasting of characters in the internal world of the client, often the problem presented as an individual challenge is also an organisational dilemma. Is experiencing extreme stress when working on the pathway responsible for ensuring an organisational target is met (four hour waiting lists for example) a story of an individual or a story of the organisation? Is worrying about the impact of a new role when you are required to make the transition without enough training and support an individual or an organisational problem? Is feeling distressed because you fear that the emerging culture has left you behind, an individual or an organisational problem? Is it an individual or an organisational problem if you feel tired because the recommendation of a certain drug may be challenged by cost implications and then you worry about what this means for a) your relationship with the patient and b) your idea of what a doctor is, does, and should be?

Maybe the people who don't seek psychological support in these complex contexts are more resilient? Or maybe the people who come to see the psychologist are more attuned to their emotional life? Maybe they are simply in touch with the fear that organisational priorities and clinical quality sometimes feel as if they are pulling against each other in the current healthcare context, a fear that many others are working hard to keep out of view? Perhaps many staff are trying to avoid becoming overly troubled by the knowledge that the culture in which they began working is not the culture in which they now find themselves?

The many ways in which the wheels kept turning, constantly repositioning staff and exposing them to new levels of organisational reality, was kept in mind in understanding referrals and also used to make sense of the organisation that was sending them through. Paying attention to fluctuations in individual and organisational experience contributed to the development of the therapeutic approach and the evolution of the role within the organisation.

A tale of crisis and change

Fight or flight: avoiding splitting and managing transition

One young manager was referred to the service after tendering her resignation. She had been recently promoted to a managerial job with an excellent performance record but was finding the new role difficult. She judged herself to have failed and wanted to leave. A colleague suggested that she saw the psychologist first.

It emerged in the first meeting with the psychologist that in many ways she was unprepared for the reality of balancing operational and strategic work, and the emotional complexity that this new role introduced into her relationships with colleagues. The role was both busy and challenging and her response to the stress she was experiencing was to internalise and suppress it. She had to implement difficult decisions, manage colleagues much older than her who had previously been friends, and she was required to say no a lot. By the time she was referred she was determined to resign and tried to use the first session to give a detailed account of her incompetence. She was extremely distressed and humiliated by all her tears in this session and by her inability to keep her vulnerability hidden. She had failed, other people didn't cry, she was unable to make transitions without collapsing, she didn't want people to see what an emotional woman she was. This was her chance and she had blown it.

Her solution was to withdraw, accept the verdict of her harsh internal jury and plan to eventually resume her career in an organisation where she had not humiliated herself. By rejecting the space to consider alternative explanations of what was happening to her she was paradoxically colluding with a one-dimensional understanding of work life. By trying to stay in control, she was expressing her strength in a harmful way. By denying the complexity she so desperately needed to appreciate in order to take up this role with authority and a more realistic understanding of the relationship between vulnerability and strength, she was ignoring the role played by the organisation in the experience she had just had.

But she didn't really want to leave, and avoiding the collusion allowed us to create a space. Through gentle challenges and exploration of the way in which the role had been designed and set up, a consideration of the limited induction and support she had had, and the perfect storm created by this context and her own unrealistic expectations, she was able to develop a new understanding of what had happened and a different relationship to her own vulnerability. By accepting rather than rejecting her emotional response she became able to think. The need to blame, either herself, or the organisation, was reduced. The thinking space allowed us to neutrally consider the many factors both individual and organisational that had contributed to her experience.

She returned successfully to the role where she soon flourished. Alongside the therapeutic work there was an opportunity, with her permission, to feed back to management an assessment of what might have helped organisationally to avoid this problem from occurring. A quick pickup and a good referral prevented this woman from leaving with a very negative view of herself.

This outcome would have also allowed the department to stay blind to the unhelpful way in which they had designed this role. Both would have been costly omissions, at an emotional and financial level. This same approach was taken with the other example above, of a nurse experiencing extreme anxiety when moved from a ward to a clinic-based job.

The predominance of linear and self-critical thinking

Many individuals presented like these women at the first session of therapy, expressing a belief that they were coping much less well than other staff in the hospital. The way in which they told their story suggested a harshness in the way they related to themselves and a strong tendency to "either/or" thinking. Either I am a good or bad doctor or manager. Either I am a strong and resilient nurse in control of my feelings or I am tearful and not worthy of this job. Throughout their stories there were hints of a belief that others in the organisation didn't struggle as they do, wouldn't need to see a psychologist, and that ultimately it was due to some personal failing that they did. This tendency to explain difficulties at an individual level was held both by individuals who self referred and managers who referred staff. Rather than considering whether the design of a job, the content of the work, or the way in which individuals and teams were supported and managed, was significant to the experience of stress, the individual was more often seen as the source of the problem.

This creates both intolerable burdens and a denial of the reality of working life and its emotional complexity, which needs a much more nuanced consideration of the many interlinked factors that may lead individuals to become stressed and unhappy at work in healthcare. The tendency to focus on the individual rather than the system is colluded with at many levels, including national initiatives to improve the health of healthcare staff which often target interventions at them rather than at the design and resourcing of their work, and the systems and structures in which they work. It is of course just a heartbeat away from blaming staff for a situation that may in fact be harming them. This feeds into the already existing default position in which rather than seeing the courage required to withstand and persevere with difficult work, moments of vulnerability can be seen as evidence of lack of fitness for organisational life and experienced as either a call to leave, or to become more robust.

Challenging "either/or" thinking, taking a systemic perspective, creating a sense of acceptance, and reflecting on the reasons why an individual may find it easier to be compassionate to patients but not to themselves, were all important areas of psychology work. While hoping to increase self-awareness, the work also aimed to develop a more critical understanding of the context in which the work is taking place. The need for an organisation-wide recognition of the emotionally challenging nature of the work, and the harm caused by responding to difficulty by attributing blame, became more and more obvious as the psychology service developed. The benefits of finding a way in which staff could become more compassionate towards themselves and their colleagues, in order to keep working effectively, grew clear. The value of creating a position in which staff could see the many ways in which the challenges of the work and the systems in which it takes place influenced behaviour, created problems, and produced distress was apparent. Perhaps making this complexity more visible could increase understanding, reduce "either/or" thinking, and develop a more realistic relationship to the experience of difficulty.

Considering the significance of the relationship to help (Fredman & Reder, 1996)

Running a psychology service in a work context one quickly becomes aware of the ability of individuals' experiencing very high (clinical) levels of distress to continue to work and function successfully in role. Sometimes this can be at the expense of their non-work identity and personal life. The fine line between functional and dysfunctional coping, and the distinction between healthy resilience and unhelpful defences, is an interesting one to reflect on, but the function of work to provide meaning, stability, and structure at a time of personal crisis, or while living with an ongoing, chronic, and recurring condition (depression for example), is very apparent in a work psychology service.

So at the time of a new referral accessing the service one of the key questions to consider was "Why now?" What alignment of individual and organisational realities was disrupted enough for someone to consider that he could not manage his emotional experience on his own? The service aimed to respond to this rupture by creating an acceptance of the felt need for help (before, during, and after it was received). Attention was paid to what aspects of a client's emotional life he felt comfortable with, and which elements he was hoping to leave behind in the psychologist's office. Often individuals would attend in crisis and it seemed as if they were hoping to leave the extreme distress behind so that they could return to the workplace with their vulnerability hidden away and being safely looked after by someone else.

While some clients would be able to productively receive the solace and comfort of a different space, others could only intermittently and reluctantly enter into a relationship with psychology in which integration of all aspects of their experience was possible. Their sense of fragmentation, apparent in the difficulties that they were experiencing in their life and exacerbated by the often fragmented nature of hospital work, could also be enacted in the way in which they related to the service. The need to keep vulnerable and more powerful aspects of themselves separate would persist and be maintained by organisational culture. Recognising that the way in which clients' relationship to help is expressed may be an enactment of their attachment style and ultimately of their relationship to themselves, provided an opportunity to consider with them the meaning of the way in which they were addressing their difficulties. Considering the strategies they used to move towards and away from their own distress and vulnerability over time provided opportunities to focus on their resources, flexibility, and creativity, and to slowly nudge them towards finding a way to accept all aspects of their experience.

The work, then, was planned with reference to many contexts—the relationship to self, to work, and to the organisation. It aimed to reposition an individual in relation to his experience and to his own sense of crisis and anxiety. Allowing clients to dictate the pacing of the therapy in response to the needs of their job—to leave and then return to therapy later for example—enabled the work to mirror the texture of organisational life and to model flexibility. This approach aimed to offer therapy within an appreciation of the sometimes unforgiving nature of organisational life. It conveyed confidence that individuals within their social networks have the ability to manage pain and to sustain themselves alone, even when struggling. In this way distress and anxiety could, where appropriate, be normalised and internal resources become more visible. The psychology service was offered as a creative and flexible resource that brought an extra dimension to individual and organisational life, but could also adapt and be responsive to context. There was also an implicit recognition of the potential for a cathartic consultation to take place in different settings. Sometimes a piece of therapeutic work could take place in an unexpected and surprising way.

A tale of forgetting about yourself

The loneliness of management and the importance of one step backwards

In July 2005 terrorist suicide bombers attacked London. Fifty-two people died and 700 were injured on Tube trains and buses. The major incident policy was activated throughout London and the hospital was put on standby to receive casualties. Throughout the day it was unclear how many people were injured and trapped underground and there were rumours of thousands of casualties. The hospital held its breath. The Accident and Emergency department (A&E) and operating theatres were cleared to make way for the injured as relatives started to arrive and casualties were admitted. In the end the numbers seen were, mercifully, much lower than those originally expected.

In many ways London had been waiting for this awful day and there had been much contingency planning beforehand. Afterwards the day was reviewed and the major incident policy was revised. The psychologist was asked to amend and develop the sections of the policy related to staff support and trauma debriefing. As part of this work she arranged to meet with members of the team responsible for managing all operational aspects of the day. One of these was a very senior manager who would have been perceived to be authoritative, direct, and fearless in her management style and who had been central to the smooth running of the hospital on that day. The meeting took place in her office and the psychologist brought some new drafts of the policy to discuss with her.

Ten minutes into the discussion and without warning the manager broke down in tears and wept as she recalled the day. She was very distressed and the psychologist was completely taken by surprise to see the depth of the emotion and her anguish. When she became calmer she was able to explain what had triggered the tears. Because the hospital, like all the London hospitals, was expecting large numbers of casualties, the focus was on fast-tracking them on admission and doing speedy triage. All casualties were moved very swiftly through A&E which then braced itself for the next cohort—but they never arrived. And this manager felt grief-stricken because she felt that in hindsight she had not attended to these first admissions with enough care. She had not spent time with them, touched them, reassured them, and asked them how they were. She had instead stayed firmly in role and ensured that everyone on the shop floor did their job and that the admissions were dispatched as quickly as possible to the most appropriate part of the hospital. She had implemented the policy perfectly but now she felt that she had let these patients down, and that she had not treated them with compassion. It seemed as she spoke that what she was expressing as a loss for them was a loss for her too, the opportunity to express her humanity in the face of trauma.

Within the meeting there was time and space to reflect this back to her, to consider how the role created an internal split, exacerbated because of the trauma, where the instinct to draw close to the patients had to be overridden so that the role could be taken up effectively to ensure that the needs of *all* patients were kept in mind and the department operated effectively. Without space to release the emotion and energy that had been needed to maintain the divide between instinct and required performance, the emotional experience became overwhelming, as did the risk of self-criticism and judgement. The sad outcome of all of this unexpressed emotion was that a feeling of failure was obscuring the success that had been achieved.

The meeting allowed the raw personal experience underneath a very controlled and successful public performance to be expressed. But it also allowed for a real appreciation of the influence of role on the extent to which individuals perceive that they have permission to feel and to express emotion and how little time there is at senior management level to reveal, discuss, and share feelings of vulnerability, fear, and loss. It highlighted the need to have space to acknowledge the personal impact of a major trauma and the high cost of being responsible for ensuring that a hospital delivers a service, at a time of high anxiety, and on a day when everyone was frightened.

And it hinted at the possibility of a deeper weight being carried by senior managers: the burden of worrying about the implications of a possible disconnect between the imperative to deliver care quickly and efficiently, and the ability to provide the reassurance and kindness that anxious patients need. This was also one of many meetings at this time where, by virtue of what the psychology role symbolised, a very different conversation to the one expected was able to take place behind closed doors. The need to keep this conversation private and confidential was unspoken but clear. The value of being able to create more public spaces for this kind of conversation was clear too.

The work of the psychologist became more visible around this time and the service started to move further into the organisation. The psychologist was asked to sit on the clinical governance committee and report on staff well-being. The psychologist and human resources set up a mediation service jointly. The psychologist was called in to debrief after trauma. Each piece of work exposed the psychologist to the creative, rich work that was taking place in the hospital, and at the same time the very difficult challenges which the organisation was facing. Moving from clinical to organisational work and back again the psychologist learnt to switch roles, to face both ways, and became more curious about how to create a space in which it was possible to keep individual and organisational realities in mind at the same time.

The need for a restoration of hope

At the heart of the psychological work there was an awareness of the need for sensitivity to the importance of hope in working life. Feeling restricted in the ability to fully fulfil the role that one has chosen at work in the way that blends personal and professional values, worrying about being able to provide the best care possible, feeling that the relationships with patients and families are being disrupted by organisational changes—all of these worries can leave healthcare staff feeling pessimistic and fearful.

Many healthcare staff are finding it harder to feel hopeful in their work as they sense themselves to be less contained[4] by the organisations in which they work and feel less sure of the compatibility between clinicians' values and the financial imperatives shaping healthcare now. Organisational changes to the delivery of care are seen by many to be diminishing the hopes and ideals with which they began their career. The difficulty of keeping clinical and organisational priorities aligned is pervasive at all levels of the system. Often these layers of tension are invisible and trickle into roles and teams in unexpected and unseen ways.

---

[4]Containment refers to the psychological process by which through appropriate support an individual feels that his emotional experience is manageable: neither overwhelming in its intensity or needing to be denied, but able to be named, digested, and understood. The repeated, successful experience of positive containment builds individual confidence in the ability to manage emotional experience when alone.

A tale of replacing solutions with understanding

Finding space to resist the impulse to act and react: withstanding organisational ambiguity

Over the period of a couple of months a number of physiotherapists contacted the psychologist through a variety of routes. Some junior staff were referred because they were tearful and stressed at work and there were ongoing conflicts between two teams. Senior members of the service asked for some coaching and consultancy and a number of middle managers (with part clinical/part managerial roles) self-referred. The physiotherapy service treats a wide range of problems, many with a psychological component. Interventions are physical and focus on the body but strong emotions are being absorbed from the patient at the same time. That was one context within which this sudden pressure on the psychology service to see physiotherapists was considered. The other context was that at the time there was a possibility that some aspects of the physiotherapy service would be put out to competitive tender. Even a well established, evidence based, and highly regarded clinical service was at risk from a competitor who could undercut its prices.

How could this anxiety and high emotion be managed? What was the best response from a psychology service feeling pressured and tugged at by clinicians at all levels of this clinical hierarchy? The psychologist was beginning to hear different versions of the same stories repeated in various clinical sessions and starting to feel fragmented and unable to contain the secrets and the worry, perhaps as the physiotherapists themselves were. This clearly wasn't sustainable.

It was decided to offer two learning sets to the middle management physiotherapists. The aim was to create an opportunity for containment and to reflect on their relationship to current work and organisational experiences. The hope was that this would impact positively on other parts of the system given the pivotal role that this group of managers had. The psychologist facilitated the sets to encourage participants to listen to each others' stories, to consider the personal and professional meaning of the challenges they faced and the emotions raised by the experiences discussed, and to try to help them to process and digest experiences without "shooting from the hip". What was most striking in the early learning sets was how difficult the physiotherapists found it to listen without rescuing. Each story would be offered a solution almost before it was finished. Each difficult emotion was made better by colleagues eagerly reassuring each other that they had done their best, each "mistake" soothed and smoothed over. There was a rush to action, a focus on learning and doing, a sense of time urgency, and a need to "tidy up".

Through the learning sets the physiotherapists were encouraged to resist the temptation to rescue and to offer solutions to each others' problems when they were discussed. It seemed that it might be beneficial to simply help them to stay still, to avoid the movement towards action, to sit with difficulty without resolving problems or absolving each other. Helping them to bear witness to each other without rushing to take responsibility allowed over time for the experiences to be digested with more depth and for meaning to be considered through the emotional experience of stillness rather than the behavioural experience of busyness and action. The aim was to develop a sense of inner authority and confidence that a difficult experience could be managed, held, and understood. The psychologist modelled this and aimed through the modelling and the creation of this experience to convey, rather than speak about, the possibility of a different relationship to "urgent" experience. The hope was that over time the group would develop skills and insights to do this with their staff.

In some ways this was providing an intervention that was countercultural. Physiotherapists are trained to be active problem solvers and doers. Creating an experience that moved in the opposite direction to this well embedded and useful skill set provided an opportunity for them to connect to a different type of intelligence and knowing. It aimed to link intellectual (every problem must have a solution) and emotional (some problems have to be lived with, some solutions aren't obvious and need space to emerge, some problems have no solution) experience. After the ten-month action learning set the physiotherapists reported lower levels of stress, and the high rate of referral to the psychology service had reduced.

The importance of relationship and creativity

While clients using the psychology service often had significant difficulties and battled their own self-criticism, many continued to work although they were suffering. So they were often asked:

"I know how bad you have been feeling—how did you manage to get out of bed—how did you get to work today?"

And invariably they would say it was their patients who brought them to work. Senior staff who had been promoted to management jobs and who were suffering were sometimes surprised to realise how much they were missing clinical work.

When we discussed what it was about the clinical work that helped or was missing there seemed to be two elements: the opportunity to be creative and to be in relationship with others. Healthcare work provides opportunities for a unique blending of emotional and intellectual resources to treat illness and protect health by developing a healing relationship. And within that relationship to have the opportunity to stay alive to change, to draw together all the evidence about an illness and its treatment (often rapidly changing) and to combine this with knowledge of an individual and his family, their hopes for the future and the quality of life they want to have. This rewarding process sustains individuals working in healthcare, as much as it does good for patients. It provides opportunities for intimacy and to make a huge difference in people's lives. Within these powerful relationships there are opportunities for creativity, and chances to think quickly, to craft sensitively, and to get immediate feedback, all very rewarding aspects of work.

The psychological work that was done aimed to encourage recognition of the reciprocal nature of this relationship, and an appreciation that it is the opportunity to be creative within a relationship that is rewarding. Feeling let down, disappointed, blocked in that endeavour is depleting to the healthcare professional. As is denying the reciprocity. Therapeutic work enabled clients to consider the hopes and needs that they brought into their work, the intimacy and intensity of it, and the way in which staff emotions could reverberate with those of the patients and families they worked with. It highlighted the importance of staying aware of the boundary between the personal and the professional, between staff needs and patients' needs, in the development of creative and productive relationships at work.

Tales of creativity and courage

Safe working at the interface—the power and the helplessness of it all

Over time the psychologist was invited to work with new teams and services led by innovative and dynamic clinicians. One of these services was PARRT, the Patient at Risk and Resuscitation Team. This is a team of highly skilled clinicians who work on the wards with very sick patients or patients who suddenly start to deteriorate. The aim is to bring a form of intensive care to the bedside to reduce the need for admission to intensive care or to begin the work that would continue on arrival at intensive care. A key part of this work is to support ward teams in a facilitative way to help manage the anxiety which quickly builds when a patient becomes acutely unwell, without deskilling ward staff. That is, to be seen as helpful, rather than critical, experts. The work is intensive, rewards those who like to see quick results and work with an adrenalin rush, and requires the ability to act quickly without overly frightening patients, staff, and relatives: a complex skill set. Like many specialist teams in healthcare it requires self-motivated autonomous individuals capable of working as part of a team but prepared to work alone, often at unsociable hours. It is a complex mix of lonely responsibility and flexible joint working.

The manager of the service asked the psychologist to do team development work, which then led to the regular provision of team supervision. At the time three different components of the team: the day, night, and resuscitation teams were all merging. The aim of the work was to create a shared identity and sense of team coherence through facilitating recognition of areas of common purpose, of the value of using interdependencies productively, and of managing differences proactively.

Over time this was a role taken with other teams too. Teams led by wise, innovative clinicians able to compete and establish groundbreaking services in a macho healthcare context. They were intuitively aware of the importance of knitting into the fabric of their services an acknowledgement that the work has an emotional cost. They were determined that the work organisation would help the team bear the cost.

These team sessions involved simply opening a space and watching and noticing together what emerged. Sometimes it would be stories of loneliness. Being in the hospital on call at night and having the buck stop with you about a life and death decision. Making the decisions as a clinician with the background of team support, but thinking afterwards about the personal loneliness of it; and the loneliness for patients and families too, facing death in the small hours of the morning; absorbing the family's uncertainty about what might happen next, how much hope and reality is left over to save them with, and how very strange it is to have your fate rely on a stranger.

Other times it would be stories of power. Members of the team would describe acting alone with authority, gathering together all the fear, and making risky decisions seem obvious and feel safe. All the time being perched right on the edge of the delicate balance between hope and uncertainty. Bearing the brunt of the need for answers: the patient's, the family's, the ward teams' needs. Or stories of heroism. Knowing that quick action and quick thinking had made a difference but now that the crisis had successfully passed, reeling from the extent of the power they had.

The sessions allowed these stories to be told, without pressure and without a need for certainty. They allowed for a meander, ensured each storyteller was able to stop at each pause and intake of breath, and consider where the weight was and where the lightness. What was the theme? What was the crucial aspect of the experience for them? The creativity that the clinician had drawn on, the humour and care that colleagues had contributed, the support provided by the team, could be pointed at and acknowledged. The aim was to create space within which to observe the unpredictable kaleidoscope of elements that made up the work at the edge of life and death that the clinicians carried out with superb humane professionalism. It seemed that they craved the intimacy and the adrenalin but had to disown them to keep moving through the flow of the work without being overwhelmed. The sessions allowed them to digest this experience, to make the power and the powerlessness seem more manageable, and to acknowledge the feelings of vulnerability which they provoked.

The relationship to work

Another relationship important to conceptualising the problems seen in the psychology service was the relationship to work. That is what was the meaning of work in this individual's life and how did it coexist with other key relationships, with partners, family, and friends for example? What place does it have and what does it represent to them? Work fulfils many needs. It functions as an expression of hope, values, and identity. It provides experiences of competence, control, autonomy, and belonging, and enables individuals to develop skills, authority, and confidence. Healthcare work allows individuals to save lives, to express care, compassion, and tenderness, to alleviate pain and fear, and to make people better. Work provides opportunities to receive praise and to be admired, as well as to provide financially for oneself and others. All these dimensions indicate why experiencing emotional difficulties in a work context that disrupt these possibilities can be so distressing and challenging. For some individuals work fulfils deeper needs and may be used as a way of managing a shaky sense of self and an underlying difficulty in regulating self-esteem. The relationship with work may help to retain a sense of coherence and control. Work successes can help to solidify a shakier sense of self-worth. Work crises can be extremely threatening.

Ultimately, though however an individual decides to express the relationship to work, everyone needs to know that what is inside him can lead to something tangible, good, and useful outside him. Erickson's apt description of the ingredients for good health, "to love and to work", resonates powerfully when providing psychology services to work settings. Losing the ability to work effectively impacts on the ability to love, that is, to be creative and express tenderness towards self and others. It threatens aspects of personal life. Having difficulties at home impacts on the ability to work. Perhaps it is the relative balance of the two, the extent to which needs are met in each area, that will determine the place and meaning of work in individual lives. The therapy provided as part of the psychology service created a place to explore this, to consider the arenas people needed to have available to them, in order to cast and direct their own inner theatre in a way that protected their emotional health and safeguarded their ability to work and to love.

Exits: disappointment, harm, and hope in organisational life

In one year 30 per cent of people seen in the psychology service were leaving the organisation. Was this a good or bad thing? A proper use of this limited resource? There is a story told earlier concerned with the importance of helping someone to stay, but it seemed also important to help people leave well. People leave for many reasons. Some of them are positive. To go to a promotion, to make a career change, or simply because life moves on, families change location, priorities shift. But each year some people also used the service to digest the experience of not fitting the culture any more. Things had changed and there was no longer a place for them and their role. Organisational change and the turning of the wheel repositioned them in such a way that to stay was no longer possible.

There were sometimes toxic and bitter experiences at the heart of these stories—feelings of being rejected and hurt by the organisation. Many were torn between this feeling and a desperate need for some solace in the face of a difficult exit. Using the therapeutic space to allow for the expression of these difficult feelings, to acknowledge feelings of loss, rejection, abandonment, and fear, to process the knowledge of not belonging any more despite a huge emotional investment in the work and the organisation, seemed an important use of psychology. The importance of identifying what was left and what could still be hoped for aimed to provide inner resources for the next job. It also connected the client to positive memories of what had been achieved and experienced in this role, so easy to forget when an ending is sad or difficult.

Healthcare contexts can be tough. This reality can seem harder to digest because the work is about caring. When a toxic work experience invades a person's inner life to the point that the possibility of hope or of creative work is disrupted, it is a damaging and destructive state of affairs for the individual, but also for organisational life. The therapy aimed to provide space to consider what was possible to preserve, and what and how to let go. It developed an insight into the nature of the harm that could be done, often unconsciously, by healthcare organisations. This emerging understanding contributed to ensuring that psychology was positioned at the interface between the individual and organisation, aware of how both could cause problems for the other, but also of how both could sometimes be unrealistic about the ability of the other to make changes. And perhaps the learning from helping individuals to leave could be translated into help for those who were staying?

Exploring this possibility further developed the psychology work to take account of the impact of conscious and unconscious organisational harm. The wish for a powerful other that could make the organisation better was transformed in therapy into either concrete plans for change, or a consideration of ways to manage the disappointment and harm organisational life can cause. The hope for individuals to become different people, for conflict to disappear, and roles to be taken up with more effectiveness, that sometimes underpinned referrals made by managers, was translated into the development of training, coaching, and consultancy interventions. The aim was to provide reflective spaces within which to consider the resources and approaches needed to withstand emotional ambiguity and thus to improve the relationships to situations, individuals, and the organisation when the options for change were limited.

The context of shame and the fear of exposure

Many staff left their final session with a thank you and a hope that they would never see the psychologist again (in the nicest possible way). They said this because they knew that they probably would, in one of her other roles in the organisation, but they didn't want the "behind closed doors" work to become public. In the local village some staff who had used the service would pass by with their heads down or step into a doorway as the psychologist passed for fear of being identified as a service user. Revealing pain, distress, and a perceived inability to cope provokes the fear of exposure and is closely associated with the experience of shame. People would arrive for appointments or meetings saying "I am not a touchy feely person," in this way positioning the psychologist as something other, different, and abiding by different rules. Perhaps the psychologist put people in touch with their shame, or maybe she was seen to possess the enviable luxury of being able to feel, unlike the client who had a tough job and exterior role to maintain, and thus no time for feelings. For in the context of healthcare it can sometimes be hard to find a safe way to acknowledge the coexistence of these two possibilities, although perhaps suggesting the potential for co-existence could be useful?

Building a bridge between two worlds: incoherence and language

Healthcare work is fast-paced, organisational change is swift, organisational life is action oriented and often unforgiving and there is little time to think, or space to reflect. Being a psychologist in this context can be like being a detective under pressure, working through the fragments of stories, trying to piece them into a shape, considering which shapes will make most sense, generate the most energy, create the most hope, and make the most connections. Clients can be reluctant or eager storytellers, but time presses on regardless of their preference or how much permission they give themselves to pay attention to the invisible parts of their lives. With the speed at which they move, healthcare staff carry with them untold stories and unfinished business, some belonging to them, others to their patients. When the possibility of psychology comes into their minds, it may simply be because these stories are pressing down in some way.

The ongoing presence of the psychologist in their organisation hints at a chance to tell a story to a neutral observer, in a different way. The gap between the inner experience and outer reality may grow; the language available to bridge it becomes uncertain and some staff come to know that what they need is some help in translating. And that the release of the story may cause some pain, as well as some relief, so cannot be done alone. Perhaps because they have seen the psychologist move between two worlds, the quiet world of the therapy room, and the bustle of the organisation, they have some confidence that the translation will be sensitive and the story will be secure. They hope that it will take place in recognition of a viable connection between their inner and outer world and that the psychologist will provide safe passage between the two. In short, they hope that it is possible to dig deep and return safely.

"*I know this sounds mad ...*", it is common to hear them say, and you encourage them to continue for this is the place for the unspeakable to take shape and become an opportunity instead of a fear. At the bottom of the well of madness are feelings of love, hate, hope, fear, regret, anger, envy, loss, and disappointment. Thrown into this arena of incoherence are the private experiences of professional life, the values and needs that brought them into this work or that may be intruding on it, and an acknowledgement that in the two-way relationships that are at the heart of all healthcare, work, staff can be hurt as well as rewarded.

The aim is to help them carve out new stories in which the intimacy at the centre of healthcare work can be acknowledged, the personal needs and hopes that are brought to it can be seen, and the ways in which organisational life disappoints can be named and then managed. The hope is that complexity can be kept in view while the way forward emerges, and that energy can be drawn from understanding that ruptures can reveal helpful truths about individual and organisational realities. The wish is to help individuals and teams to stand still for a moment, listen to their own story, and watch it move them as it takes shape. In this way they will see what they have woven so far, and can be realistic about what is inside them (their own resources) and what is outside them (the organisational and work context) so that they can move forward wisely and safely.

PART II

From one culture to another
Bringing Schwartz Rounds to the UK

"I think that is all we want as human beings. That is why there are religions and philosophies. Without stories, life would be overwhelming."

Mark Rylance interview, The Daily Telegraph, *September 23, 2015*

The need for stories

A hunger you become aware of when you are suddenly fed.

Imagine a public forum where each month you could satisfy this need—or even just have it made publicly conscious ... and go away with an experience that this need for the stories that make the broken bits of emotionally full and exhausting days real and true, in both their beauty and their sadness, is not just yours but a communal need.

And that all those moments when you felt you were alone, you were only alone in the doing but never the being. That is, being a person who chose to work right on the edge of mystery and understanding, on the line between life and death. That's what the stories did for you. Your story being heard, a version of your story being told by someone else, gave the fearful smallness and the awesome powerfulness in your work a colour and a shape, a form and some flow. Resonance that connected you to others. And full stops that gave you space to step back and see, to feel and to breathe.

Implementing Schwartz Rounds in the UK: creating new spaces
and facilitating new conversations in healthcare

Introduction

By 2009 the psychology service was well established and becoming integrated with the many innovative strands of work to improve organisational culture which the hospital was developing. There were new and
exciting areas of work to become involved in and a sense of possibility
on the one hand, but a fragmented culture and many tired, stressed,
and disillusioned staff on the other. But maybe this was no different
from other UK hospitals?

The NHS: content and symbol

Nationally healthcare was also a kaleidoscope of anxiety and creativity—
the relationship between the colours, shapes, and patterns constantly
shifting. Technology and scientific developments continued to extend
the limits of what was possible diagnostically and in terms of treatment
options and patient prognosis in healthcare. But the reality of potential
and progress was pushing up against the stark problems of funding,
the demands created by the health needs of an expanding, aging
population, and the massive challenges in running financially viable
healthcare organisations.

   The political significance of the NHS, an organisation born out of
optimism and idealism and symbolically tasked with the impossible
responsibility of preserving a sense of national identity (within which
equality, generosity, and kindness are enshrined), continued to influence
the extent to which change could be overtly or covertly implemented to
address these challenges. Emotions run high in the UK in relation to
the NHS. But emotion and the business of healthcare are inextricably
connected (as ultimately its business is life, death, and survival) though
the relationship is often confused for fear of disturbing the identity that
needs to be preserved through the "idea" of the NHS.[5] Many idealistic
and nostalgic hopes are projected into it, while on a day to day basis,

---

[5]See Obholzer (1994) for a discussion of the NHS as a container of anxieties about vulnerability and death.

busy staff deliver oceans of work within which rational decisions about care need to be made in the context of both emotional and financial realities, and consequences.

The challenge of bringing together the rational and the emotional in the design, delivery, and development of healthcare services is the challenge of integration and requires that the dilemmas of modern healthcare are consistently and regularly surfaced and addressed. At every level in the system, space to think and space to feel, space to consider meaning at the same time as to respond wisely to priorities, will ensure that neither process (cognitive and emotional) can subvert or confuse the other. But the complexity of healthcare systems can make this challenge feel impossible sometimes, and so it becomes something that just gets carried, and is imperfectly resolved. And simmering below the surface is the fear that something will be lost if the balance between the two tips too much in either direction—the fear that the NHS will either become too business-like on one hand, or on the other, be unable to accept and address financial realities.

What cannot be said

Shaped by the past, pulled towards the future by innovation and creativity, in 2009 the NHS was full of anxiety, both spoken and unspoken.

How much is enough? Who can say no? What if there isn't enough to go around? How will we know when to stop intervening? How much more can healthcare systems rely on the goodwill of staff to deliver, beyond what they are contracted to do, in order that services remain viable? How much more can staff give of themselves, before they become ill? Who can speak the following truths? not everyone can be saved, everyone must die eventually, there is no perfect system, everyone is human, and sometimes we fail. Maybe healthcare provision cannot be unlimited …

And so on. The difficulty of articulating these questions publicly and consistently meant they could only be intermittently digested and considered. And in this multi-layered, partially obscured context, healthcare organisations themselves were engaged in a battle for survival of the fittest, which was escalating and intensifying. It was sweeping management up into its relentless dynamic of defensiveness and competition and further driving apart the rational and the emotional elements of the work because of the need to always appear robust enough. The dangers of fusion, when the dynamic underpinning the work (a struggle for life and health, a fight for survival) binds with the dynamic driving the system designed to deliver the work, were real and powerful. This fusion creates a context in which a collective blindness can develop, and terrible errors can begin to take place almost unnoticed (were it not for the extensive and exhausting vigilance of individual staff in their roles), until a tipping point is reached. Within this context meaning becomes elusive and the urge to blame can become irresistible.

And so the first in a series of a particular type of crisis struck about this time, with the revelation of the deficiencies in care at Mid Staffs NHS Trust (see Francis, 2013). The challenges raised by the problems it exposed quickly became formulated within a narrative of cruelty (blame always just a fingertip away) and a new policy context of compassion quickly emerged. How can we avoid cruelty and enable compassion? How can we ensure that patients are not let down in this way again? How can we improve the care patients receive? How can we *make* healthcare staff *be* more compassionate and how can we make sure that we weed out those who aren't, and punish those organisations that employ them?

The problem of integration

And so the difficulty of integration and the risk of splitting[6] persisted, the either/or narrative of cruelty and compassion developed,[7] and the triangle of patient, carer, and healthcare organisation continued. Within this triangulation one pairing is always dominant (the patient-carer relationship, or the relationship between staff and the organisation, or between the organisation and its patients, etc.) and one party's experience becomes invisible *and* potentially blameworthy, whether the patient's, the staff member's, or the organisation's. The risk posed by being unable to conceptualise this three-way relationship successfully,

---

[6]Splitting is a term from psychodynamic schools of thought and refers to an unconscious ego defence mechanism by which a fairly complex entity cannot be accepted into consciousness in its entirety because it contains aspects that are both acceptable to a person as well as unacceptable. To resolve this tension things are then seen as either "good" or "bad" because of the difficulty of holding both possibilities at the same time.

[7]Although see the Berwick report (2013) recommending ways in which to avoid the splitting and the cycle of blame.

that is, keeping all three elements simultaneously in view, can be manifested in terms of ruptures in staff well-being, patient experience, and/or organisational performance. This was the complex context that existed when Schwartz Rounds were brought to the UK.

What is a Schwartz Round?

A Schwartz Round is a monthly meeting held in a healthcare organisation where the impact of caring and the human dimensions of providing healthcare are considered. Modelled on the idea of a Medical Grand Round (held monthly in most hospitals, where a clinical team present a patient, discuss their diagnosis and treatment plan, and have an opportunity to have feedback from, and discussion with, an audience of colleagues), a Schwartz Round turns the focus onto the health professionals themselves and allows for a consideration of their own experience of providing care. Each Schwartz Round lasts for one hour and includes stories, usually of a case (or sometimes of a theme, for example, "A Patient I'll Never Forget"), told by a multidisciplinary panel. A typical panel will include three or four staff who have all been involved in the case, and who will each describe their unique experience of it and the impact that working on the case has had on them. The audience is made up of members of hospital staff all of whom (both clinical and non–clinical) are welcome to attend. Once the panel have presented, the facilitator and a medical lead (who jointly facilitate the Round) help the audience to make a connection between the stories they have just heard and similar experiences of their own. The Round then becomes a group reflection on work experience with the facilitators creating links between the stories that are shared and the work experiences of the audience, drawing out personal, professional, and organisational themes that emerge.

In the beginning was a personal story

The Rounds are named after Kenneth B. Schwartz, a Boston lawyer who died tragically of lung cancer in his forties. Before he died he wrote movingly in a magazine article (Schwartz, 1995) of the positive impact of receiving compassionate care as his prognosis became bleaker:

> Until last fall I had spent a considerable part of my career as a health-care lawyer, first in state government and then in the private

sector. I came to know a lot about health-care policy and management, government regulations and contracts. But I knew little
about the delivery of care. All that changed on November 7, 1994,
when, at age 40 I was diagnosed with advanced lung cancer. In the
months that followed, I was subjected to chemotherapy, radiation,
surgery, and news of all kinds, most of it bad. It has been a har-
rowing experience for me and for my family. And yet, the ordeal
has been punctuated by moments of exquisite compassion. I have
been the recipient of an extraordinary array of human and humane
responses to my plight. These acts of kindness—the simple human
touch from my caregivers—have made the unbearable bearable ....
If I have learned anything, it is that we never know when, how, or
whom a serious illness will strike. If and when it does, each one of
us wants not simply the best possible care for our body but for our
whole being. I am bound upon Lear's wheel of fire,[8] but the love
and devotion of my family and friends, and the deep caring and
engagement of my caregivers, have been a tonic for my soul and
have helped to take some of the sting from my scalding tears.

The article concludes:

I cannot emphasize enough how meaningful it was to me when
caregivers revealed something about themselves that made a personal
connection to my plight. It made me feel much less lonely. The rulebooks, I'm sure, frown on such intimate engagement between caregiver and patient. But maybe it's time to rewrite them ...

Within the article, however, there is an acknowledgement that this intimacy may come at a cost for the healthcare professionals and that their
training has encouraged them to create some distance between themselves and the plight of their patients in order to survive their work
in the long term. The suggestion to rewrite the rulebooks carries with
it an understanding of the need for support for staff if they are to be
encouraged to move towards, rather than away from the emotional
experience of their patients. Kenneth B. Schwartz died of lung cancer
in September 1995. Shortly before his death he founded the Schwartz
Center for Compassionate Care at Massachusetts General Hospital,

---

[8]"I am bound upon a wheel of fire that mine own tears do scald like molten lead." *King
Lear*, Act 4, Scene 7.

which is dedicated to strengthening the relationships between patients and caregivers,[9] and one of the early interventions which the Center developed were Schwartz Rounds.

Looking towards America: the solution is outside us

The Point of Care programme[10] at the King's Fund was established to improve the care patients receive in hospital and specifically to develop and support interventions that keep the patient experience at the centre of thinking about the delivery of care (Firth-Cozens & Cornwell, 2009; Goodrich & Cornwell, 2008). As their work developed they came to appreciate the crucial impact of staff experience on patients. One of the key members of the early team had begun to research interventions that could support staff in the delivery of compassionate patient care, when she came across Schwartz Rounds[11] and thought that they might transfer well to the UK.

Two initial pilot sites were identified, one being the London hospital discussed in chapter one. A medical lead and a facilitator were identified in each hospital. Both facilitators were senior psychologists who were already providing staff support services to their organisations. The teams[12] travelled together to Boston where they had an opportunity to observe a number of well-established Schwartz Rounds and to meet with experienced Schwartz Round facilitators.

Beginning the journey

We arrived late on a warm May evening and we went to our first Round the next day. This immediate, disorienting immersion in a different country was accentuated by one of the themes of this Round, which was whether or not a child was eligible for treatment in the US. The difference between the UK and US context was starkly obvious (six years later this theme is emerging in UK Rounds) in terms of access to healthcare in both countries. Culture was instantly significant and we watched the

---

[9]www.theschwartzcenter.org
[10]Founded by Dr Jocelyn Cornwell, now an independent charity called The Point of Care Foundation.
[11]Joanna Goodrich, head of evidence and learning, The Point of Care Foundation.
[12]Dr Jocelyn Cornwell, now chief executive, The Point of Care Foundation; Dr Sean Elyan, medical director and consultant in clinical oncology, Gloucester Hospitals NHS Foundation Trust; Leslie Morrison, head of health psychology, Gloucester Hospitals NHS Foundation Trust; and the author.

tension between organisational (national) reality and human instinct play out in the stories that were told. We met with the presenting team and the facilitators of this Round afterwards and were able to hear more about their work and their relationship to these stories. Over the following days we met many people working for, or with the Schwartz Center, we saw more Rounds and heard about research that was being done. We met with doctors who discussed the positive use of Rounds in medical education. We were treated to a meeting of facilitators from a wide range of Rounds who generously shared stories of their work, their creativity, and their experiences of Rounds. Their enthusiasm was infectious, the welcomes warm and generous, and the wide range of uses of Rounds apparent. We travelled back to the UK excited by the possibility of doing this work in our own organisations and wondering what we would need to do to make sure that they worked in the UK.

Conceptualising and creating a shape

One initial question that we had as we travelled to America was whether it was possible to do anything of meaning or value in such a large group? And in a group where attendance varies each time and is open to so many different staff within a hospital community. Experiencing a Round in the US suggested that (contrary to instincts) this was possible. But how? Through experiencing Rounds, through the process of learning to facilitate them, and responding to the challenges that this posed, the process of conceptualising a UK Schwartz Round developed. This process was to deepen as the implementation proceeded and this conceptualisation will be now shared with reference to relevant theory, and with examples of Rounds.

First frames: emotion and culture

There were two aspects of this trip to the US, which was replicated in the UK in both local and national implementation. First, the need to experience a Schwartz Round in order to appreciate its potential to create space for new conversations to take place and new connections to be made. That is, the need to influence through experience. The realisation that the route to implementing Schwartz Rounds had to be through emotional experience of a Round rather than rational understanding was key and at this stage yet to be fully appreciated. Of course one of the mechanisms underpinning Rounds is in fact the creation and the deepening of connections between these two realms.

The second aspect of this trip, which was to be significant in the implementation, was the importance of paying attention to culture at every level. That is, the importance of context in informing the way in which a Schwartz Round emerges in any setting, is formed, and delivers its value. The quality and impact of Rounds depends on sensitivity to context and a good understanding, and strong guidance and management, of the psychological processes at work at an individual and organisational level at each stage of this process of emergence. Culture is also important in terms of the extent to which the significance of both rational and emotional experience is acknowledged in an organisation without one or the other needing to be denied or denigrated.

A key conversation, which the team had on the way back from America, was whether this new intervention, so well established in the land of Oprah Winfrey and confessional television, would be acceptable in a UK context. This conversation was to be repeated many times when we returned to the UK and were challenged about issues such as whether people would talk openly about their feelings (or paradoxically, what would happen if these feelings got out of hand) during the implementation process in our respective hospitals.

The experience of national implementation was to provide some answers to these questions. It revealed the nuanced ways in which issues of culture (local and national) emerged in relation to Schwartz Rounds, how carefully the process of public storytelling needed to be managed in order to remain sensitive both to the demands of cultural contexts and individual emotional realities, and what a complex process can unfold within the outwardly simple structure of a Schwartz Round.

Space for translation and digestion

Schwartz Rounds can strengthen the carer/patient relationship by providing space to reflect on the cost and impact of caring. They are run in recognition of the high costs to healthcare workers of staying in daily close proximity to ill and worried patients, the cost of withstanding the emotions they absorb from patients (fear, anger, anxiety, helplessness, loss, hope, despair, for example). Rounds provide a safe space where difficult and rewarding experiences of providing care can be shared, and the resources which healthcare workers draw on to do their work can be acknowledged, explored, and celebrated. In this way over time they may help to make the more unbearable aspects of doing healthcare work bearable (Wren, 2012) and allow staff to connect to the creativity they use in their work. They also provide opportunities to surface less obvious influences on the process of providing care for example the reciprocity at the heart of the healthcare relationship. Another often invisible contributor to the emotional experience of healthcare work is the organisation within which it takes place, as hinted at in the discussion of triangulation mentioned above (see page 34). The influence of this dimension on staff experience was to become very evident in the UK implementation process.

Beginning in a new context

Schwartz Rounds were piloted in two NHS Trusts (Royal Free London NHS Foundation Trust and Gloucester Hospitals NHS Foundation Trust). The question of whether they would transfer to a UK context was convincingly answered by both high attendance and the enthusiastic and positive way in which staff on both sites engaged with them. The initial pilot study concluded that the "two English Trusts have shown that Schwartz Center Rounds can transfer to a UK NHS context. Rounds appear to be valued by staff at all levels and are firmly established in the two pilot trusts, providing a good foundation for their future spread" (Goodrich & Levenson, 2011). The King's Fund began to roll out Rounds to some other hospitals and also to hospices. In 2013 the UK Department of Health provided funding for a national rollout of Rounds and the Point of Care Programme became an independent charity, The Point of Care Foundation.[13] The author began to work for the charity, leading on the development of both the mentoring that was provided to organisations as they set up and began Rounds, and the national training programme for facilitators and medical leads (Wren, 2015). The remainder of this chapter reflects on this experience and proposes a conceptual understanding of the processes that were observed as organisations and individuals were supported and developed to implement Rounds safely and creatively.

Implementation: keeping micro and macro in mind

The success of Schwartz Rounds in an organisation depends on two things: what happens within the hour of the Round, and what happens outside the hour: that is, the creation of an infrastructure that will

---

[13]www.pointofcarefoundation.org.uk

develop the Round and sustain the facilitators to choose, prepare, and use stories that have clinical and organisational relevance. Their ability to wisely position themselves to enable links to be drawn between micro and macro level experience is key to maintaining the relevance of the Round over time.

To support facilitators and medical leads to hold true to the purpose of the Rounds, and to link the Rounds to organisational structure, a steering group meets monthly and provides executive level support and endorsement of the process. The steering group is made up of senior and junior staff from across the organisation who represent all staff groups. They help with choosing cases and identifying topics to be covered in Rounds. They also debrief individual Rounds and consider important quality issues such as safety and confidentiality. They regularly promote Rounds and increase their reach within the organisation by targeting their respective work areas to identify and offer cases for the Round. The steering group has a key role in helping the organisation to manage the implementation process.

Positioning and holding

However the steering group are internal to the organisation's culture, bound by its rules and dynamics, keen for Rounds to succeed in this culture but acting often to maintain it, while it can be argued that the process of Schwartz Round implementation is in many ways counter-cultural. Good Rounds shift an organisation and its workers away from their default position of urgent action, reaction, and problem solving to an hour of stillness and slowness. Within this still place culture can be noticed and observed and the influences on professional and personal behaviour can be commented on. The facilitators and medical leads are key to the subtle process of positioning of the Round. It is their role[14] to help the steering group and the organisation resist the pull to action, and to notice and observe "hidden rules" and gently draw them back to witnessing, and to considering the meaning of staff and organisational experiences. At the early stages of implementation they need help to do this effectively and to manage the impact of the organisation's culture on their development and facilitation of the Round. As well as the active

---

[14]*Facilitators* is used from now on to describe both the facilitator and the medical/clinical lead.

support of the steering group, the facilitators also need a temporary hold-ing point that is external to their organisation, a platform from which to see opportunities and pitfalls more clearly and develop their own inner authority and ability to perceive the relationship between staff experi-ence and organisational context. The development of mentoring support that was an important part of the national rollout provided this exter-nal holding and a space within which to consider how organisational dynamics impacted on the facilitators and medical leads themselves.

The courage to begin: experiences of implementation

Through the implementation work the importance of this temporary exter-nal steadying was demonstrated time and time again. It quickly became apparent that the early Rounds facilitators and medical leads needed to be held safe and encouraged to hold firm, while their organisation slowly discovered how to be confident in bridging the gap between what they were hoping for (more supported staff more able to deliver compas-sionate care) and what they needed to reveal and manage (fear, anxiety, helplessness; unacceptable feelings towards patients, self, colleagues, the organisation; confronting risk and error, worry about not being good enough, worry about caring too much, etc.), in order to achieve this.

For throughout the start-up period of Rounds, organisations, while espousing their commitment to Rounds, typically throw a number of chal-lenges at the Schwartz champions. This may be because the overt link-ing of these two elements—hope and fear—by the organisation is almost impossible to achieve at the beginning of the process. Although we know intellectually that it is only in acknowledging at some level their own experience of vulnerability, with all the risks that this will involve, that staff can connect to patient vulnerability, the reality of this and the risk of dismantling individual and organisational defences feels almost unman-ageable at the beginning of establishing Rounds. So organisations need to feel their way towards managing the anxiety by firstly experiencing the containing framework of the Rounds. Then through the gradual deep-ening of understanding and development of community that takes place within the Rounds,[15] confidence grows that the processes involved are manageable as individual and organisational resources become visible in the responses to the experiences shared and a community starts to form.

---

[15]During this time there is a heavy reliance on the facilitators and medical leads to carry the risk.

The story is the engine

An important element in this process is the use of story to reveal experience in a prepared and crafted way, which allows the audience to move closer to a positive experience of *managed* exposure and a gradual acceptance of incompleteness and unfinished business. Once this process begins, anxiety which has been expressed in the following ways begins slowly to lessen:

• What happens if people get upset?
• Should we make counselling services available?
• What happens if we hear stories of poor practice?

Key to this process is the authenticity of the storytelling, and good, powerful Rounds have what one Schwartz Round facilitator[16] calls "the slide towards authenticity", where an irresistible process of storytelling draws participants together and into an honest exploration of the meaning of their work, its disappointments and challenges, its rewards, and the difficult organisational context within which it is sometimes taking place. While in touch with this authenticity the group have an opportunity to transform individual experiences of shame, anxiety, and hope into a group acknowledgement of the real nature of the work. It is fragmented and complex, peddles uncertainties, pain, loss, and failure, along with the opportunity to be creative and to experience immeasurably deep rewards, meaning, and satisfaction—just like life.

And importantly, just like life for *both* patient and caregiver. The resonance between the two realities makes individual and organisational defences vital in order for healthcare work to be done, by an individual, in the context of a relationship. Thus Rounds allow for a recognition and exploration of the undefended experience, and a temporary and structured connection to the pain and pleasure that the defences are there to manage. It is the cumulative repetition of this process through regular monthly Rounds that can allow for the development of organisational confidence that naming and witnessing the cost of the work, as well as its value, can be withstood and may ultimately strengthen resilience, connection, and understanding.

But organisations cannot be told this. They must experience it, and have space and support to process the experience. The provision of

---

[16]Raymond Chadwick, consultant clinical psychologist and Schwartz Round facilitator, South Tees NHS Foundation Trust, personal communication.

external mentoring for the start-up phase provides an opportunity for the facilitator and medical lead to do this processing, and take this risk, on behalf of the organisation. Ensuring that they had an opportunity to debrief with an external, neutral, and supportive observer, to consider with them the stories which they were being offered for Rounds and the best ways to manage the storytelling, was a key part of helping organisations to begin to integrate the various experiences that emerged as they began. This allowed organisations to embed the Rounds in a creative and constructive way that was responsive to their own unique context.

Paradox: using sensitivity to culture to allow culture to become visible

At many levels and at each stage of the implementation process, paradox is at the heart of successful Rounds implementation. This involves for example:

- Managing the desire to have slow things done quickly.
- Finding strong people to display and discuss their vulnerability.
- Managing organisational reputation while talking about feelings of failure.
- Using external support to create internal vision and authority.
- Developing a powerful space while subverting the narrative that power privileges.

The management of this paradox is pivotal and requires careful and thoughtful digestion of the challenges posed at each stage of implementation, in order to position Rounds in a way in which they will be productive and sustainable. It involves sensitively connecting elements of organisational life that may initially seem incompatible.

Once positioned effectively, without a requirement to overtly deliver on corporate, strategic, team, or individual action-oriented goals, Rounds can become a strong part of an organisation's culture, contributing in a subtle and nuanced way by repetitively deepening meaning and facilitating understanding of clinical experience and organisational life. It is the positioning of the Rounds at the interface between clinical work and staff experience, while sanctioned by organisational authority, that enables this process to occur, and protects their power and appeal. By keeping connected to the three overlapping contexts of the patient, the staff member, and the organisation without a requirement to produce an outcome for any of them, Rounds can create a space within which the triangulation of healthcare experience can be both noticed and resisted. All three layers of context can be kept in mind, in the storytelling and facilitation within each Round. To protect the quality of the Round and contribute to its silent, cumulative impact, this needs to be done in a neutral way.

By being seen as a space that is "for staff" and that will allow for a truthful exploration of authentic staff experience without the imposition of a corporate agenda, or the pressure to lean towards an ideal script or to produce an outcome, Rounds over time can create confidence that an organisation and its individuals can stay still for an hour and withstand an acknowledgement of the various realities of organisational life in healthcare. Within the boundaries needed for organisational and clini-cal safety they can nudge an organisation as close as it can safely go in a multidisciplinary space to a group recognition and acceptance of the realities of its work, the complexity of its multi-layered contexts, and the impact of both on individual staff.

Stories that seep through: what might a Round be telling us about the organisation?

The experience of developing the national training programme for medical leads and facilitators and of developing the mentoring frame-work offered rich opportunities to consider the choices that were being made nationally in relation to implementing Rounds in various organisations. Just as individual staff referred to the psychologist were always understood to be bringing a message from the organisation as well as a story of themselves, so it was helpful to stay curious about what Rounds might be saying about current organisational issues and preoccupations in different settings. How an organisation decided (consciously and/or unconsciously) to use the empty space that was the hour of a Round seemed to convey a range of messages about organisational life, priorities, and needs that were worth considering. For example, what is the current organisational emotional state, what are the rules about exposure in this organisation, what is the organisa-tion most proud of and also most ashamed of, and what stories do staff feel are not being heard?

For instance, one organisation chose to focus on errors in an early Round. The powerful stories that were told said much about the integrity and honesty of the professionals who told them, and about their emotional commitment to their work, but also seemed to suggest something about the current context, the fears and hopes that were carried in it, for the Rounds, and maybe for the organisation itself. Was there a need to confess, for example, or a worry about lack of containment? Was the organisation struggling to come to terms with some past errors? Maybe there was a desire for a public expression of shame and sorrow that also contained a hope for forgiveness? The space seemed to be being used in a confessional way. Perhaps the organisers of the Round wanted to develop their Rounds by giving permission for the unsayable to be said, to encourage longing and release to fill the vacuum and create a desire for more.

Consideration of these possibilities and of the choices that were made in relation to stories offered and accepted, as well as the stories that were chosen and told, was used as food for thought while mentoring individual facilitators and medical leads. This aimed to deepen their conceptual understanding of a Round and of the layers of meaning that were emerging through them. It also introduced the value of continuing to consider the way in which the Round was being used (and could potentially be misused) by their organisation, in order to continue to position them safely and to deepen facilitation skills. Facilitators were repeatedly encouraged to continue to consider these issues as a helpful parallel layer to pay attention to, while their organisation shaped the evolution of its Round in both conscious and unconscious ways.

Carrying risk and fragility safely: surfacing context and complexity

Panellists, then, don't just offer stories; they reveal needs, and hopes and fears. And not just their own but the organisation's too. In the mentoring facilitators were encouraged to notice themes emerging and over time decide how to surface them for consideration in the Round itself. For example, in one organisation it was notable how many panellists used the word "pride" and how it became a form of shorthand to wrap up and finish a story. "I just want to say before I finish though, how proud I was of my team," a panellist would say, regardless of the content of their tale. All the stories became shiny at the end.

But the facilitator in this organisation used the mentoring to share his shock at the level of distress he was uncovering as he walked the corridors finding stories and panellists for the Rounds. Yet the work taking place within this organisation was very tough—why was he so shocked? The rules about what must stay hidden, and the importance of organisational reputation, were playing out both within and around the Rounds. The wider NHS context, within which the fear of organisational and clinical failure and the need to compete is real and active, seemed significant. The need for the organisation to be seen to be successful and the work a source of pride, the uncertainty about what can be said (and where), were creating this splitting of experience and the slide into triangulation where staff experience must stay invisible, to maintain organisational reputation. Within this manifestation of a three-way split, only organisational pride and successful patient outcomes could be kept in view. The mentoring aimed to help facilitators consider how to resist the triangulation and keep all three levels of experience in mind while managing at times the group or organisation's need to split off or deny one level of experience.

There are many ways in which meaning can be surfaced and mentoring aimed to develop courage, authority, and a calibrated sense of pacing in facilitators. Once facilitators learned how to stay sensitive to process within the group itself, then they could pair this with their knowledge of the organisation to decide over time how best the complexity underpinning the stories that were brought to Rounds could be noticed. One way might be through managing the group's response to the stories that were told. In this way, truths could be named through a group acknowledgement of organisational and clinical realities, through community witnessing rather than in one voice or story. An organisation could watch themes emerge rather than be told truths. The story could pull the group towards the unsayable. The facilitation could help it to be received. A passive, softer process of emergence could create a new relationship to experience within which compassion and understanding were possible and no single person could be blamed for speaking out of turn.

Connecting the incompatibles: resetting through unexpected couplings

In this example above the relief in being honest, ("This work is hard and distressing") balanced with the recognition that reputation is important to the survival of the organisation, could through skilled and neutral facilitation lead to a helpful and creative exploration of the double nature of organisational life in healthcare. This could create the possibility for a

sort of psychological "settling" that may be very helpful in staff relationships to their work, their organisation, and ultimately their patients.

In considering the multiple realities that are pushing up against the
boundary of a Round we could consider the words of Seamus Heaney
(1995):

> Yet there are times when a deeper need enters, when we want
> the poem to be not only pleasurably right but compellingly wise,
> not only a surprising variation played upon the world, but a
> re-tuning of the world itself. We want the surprise to be transitive
> like the impatient thump which unexpectedly restores the picture
> to the television set, or the electric shock which sets the fibrillat-
> ing heart back to its proper rhythm … we want to be … true to
> the impact of external reality and … sensitive to the inner laws of
> the poet's being.

This quote, written though it is to explain what we need from poetry,
sums up most beautifully both the settling process that can occur within
a good Round, and also the tension between individual and organisational reality in any context. Creating an authentic Round that is sensitive to delicate and complex inner experience and also realistic about the
harsh context in which healthcare is delivered may have the potential
to enable staff to name and withstand both realities. It can reduce the
space between them and the likelihood of denial of either reality, a state
in which problems can emerge, both for individuals and organisations.

Conducting the process: linking story to clinical and organisational reality to create a new space

So the empty space of the Schwartz Round and how it is used can tell
us much about organisational rules and hidden meanings, about the
denial of distress and the management of staff experience within organisations, about shame and hope, all of which make up the rich canvas
within which the facilitators work. It also has the potential for a productive resettling. It can be a potent space within which creative reparation
can emerge, allowing clinicians and organisations to come full circle in
their understanding of themselves, each other, and their organisation.
Facilitation is key to this process.

The implementation process helped to shape our understanding of the
facilitation task, and how to connect it to the organisational and cultural

context. By continuing to unravel the meaning of our experience at each stage of the implementation process, and to position facilitators in ways that would create possibilities for productive storytelling within their organisations, we had begun to create new spaces for different conversations to take place in healthcare organisations throughout the country. Our journey to the US and back (and then out again to many hospitals and hospices in the UK), had brought clarity about how to safely bring this unique space to this new culture. We could now describe what needed to be done. We could consider how to respond to the possibility of splitting in the positioning of the Rounds, which the organisational contexts had the potential to produce. We knew the importance of harnessing facilitators' creativity and developing their authority to ensure that Rounds processes cultivated a realistic sense of compassion for staff, a necessary prerequisite for the provision of compassionate care (see Wren, 2014).

Part III of this book narrows the focus to describe the experience of learning to do this in just one organisation. But here beforehand is a description of the pivotal process of facilitation, the hinge on which the whole enterprise of creating new pathways to connection swings, and the key skill in the process of containment that underpins a productive Round.

Using their knowledge of the organisation, allowing their mentor to initially bridge the gap between external and internal authority, drawing on their steering group to feed them organisational experiences, hopes, and fears, the medical lead and the facilitator choose cases, prepare panellists, and help craft stories to be told in public.

Once the Round has begun they are then the visible conductors of the process. The orchestration has begun outside the Round through the identification of the themes and issues raised by the stories and the gentle, focussed process of shifting the storyteller away from attention to the patient as the central organising element of the story, and towards a curiosity about the storyteller's own experience: personal, professional, and organisational. Now in the Round the facilitators use their learning from this process to manage the flow of the discussion and ensure all three contexts (staff, patient, organisation) are linked to the stories, and experiences, the thoughts and the dynamics that occur in the Round both within individuals and within the group.

Over time they learn to use their own experience of the process of panel preparation and facilitation to guide them towards each next, new step in facilitation where rational and emotional experience have equal permission to emerge, and can be noticed and coexist, remarked upon and digested, moved towards and away from. That process of deepening meaning, shifting over and back to earlier themes, linking micro and macro level experience, speeding up or slowing down the music, and stitching in a story that was present in the preparation but temporarily forgotten, comes later.

In the early Rounds the facilitators just need strong, confident arms to momentarily hold back the national context, the organisational structures, the inner and outer rules, that dictate relationships and behaviour and allow a story to be told which speaks to the group by simply being the story of what they do, and where they are. By simply being the story of who they are.

Schwartz Rounds: content, symbol, container

And so in this way stories of working in the UK healthcare at this time began to be told and the shape of this new space began to emerge in a different culture and was enthusiastically taken up and used. And though the content and topic of each Round varied each month, in each organisation, throughout the country, a number of common themes threaded their way into the stories and pushed into the Rounds in spoken and unspoken ways:

How much is enough? Who can say no? What if there isn't enough to go around? How will we know when to stop intervening? How much more can healthcare systems rely on the goodwill of staff to deliver, beyond what they are contracted to do, in order that services remain viable? How much more can staff give of them, before they become ill? Who can speak the following truths?: not everyone can be saved, everyone must die eventually, there is no perfect system, everyone is human, and sometimes we fail. Maybe healthcare provision cannot be unlimited …

And through training and mentoring facilitators developed skills and understanding to hold the unsayable sensitively, to ensure that the shape and form of this new intervention would emerge creatively and responsively so that meaning could be surfaced at a safe and productive pace for each individual organisation.

Separating the dancer from the dance

Using systemic thinking to implement a new intervention

… Labour is blossoming or dancing where
The body is not bruised to pleasure soul.
Nor beauty born out of its own despair,
Nor blear-eyed wisdom, out of midnight oil.
O chestnut-tree, great-rooted blossomer,
Are you the leaf, the blossom or the bole?
O body swayed to music, O brightening glance,
How can we know the dancer from the dance?

W. B. Yeats, Amongst School Children, *1928*

Separation and integration: linking private and public experiences in healthcare settings

The development of the psychology service described in Part I of this book had provided an insight into the reality of working in a hospital, providing care, managing staff, and managing oneself, in order to stay effective and cope with an often overwhelming level of work demands, operational, physical, and emotional. It had also highlighted frameworks and positions that were most useful in ensuring that the service matched the pace and the style of hospital work, staying close enough to be credible but offering something different.

Experience of psychology service provision had demonstrated the need for safe spaces where real experience could be shared without fear or shame, and where conflict and difficulty could be normalised. It showed the value of allowing staff time simply to pay attention to their own emotional life without judging or denying it. It appeared that this new intervention could provide opportunities to do all these things while enabling private conversations to now take place in public spaces. The benefits of combining narrative psychology and systemic thinking to provide a conceptual framework within which to hold this process sensitively, in order to balance the performance element with the management of the emotional realities that would emerge and be exposed, was quickly to become apparent.

The opportunity to implement this new intervention arose at the time that the psychology service was well established and becoming linked to the developing work on culture change. The process of implementation became a catalyst, which deepened and integrated many ongoing interventions aiming to improve staff experience and organisational culture. The ways in which the stories were crafted, performed, and held enabled prescient clinical and organisational themes to emerge for consideration in a new non–hierarchical forum. The moves that were made at each stage to stay responsive to culture, risk, and hope in order to craft private experience for a public telling will now be described.

Using emerging meaning to craft stories

In essence Rounds link narrative psychology and reflective practice in a large group organisational space. They are a subtle mixture of the processing of work experience, and of storytelling and performance.

They work both literally and symbolically to create opportunities for new ways of thinking and talking about work both within and outside the hour. In a large group setting they both provide and suggest a new way of relating to the experience of working in healthcare. And they are also an opportunity to develop a shared community exploration of the emotional undertow, of healthcare work, the impact of its complexity on individuals and on teams.

Getting Started

The early work involved forming the team. They were a psychologist (the author), a renal medicine consultant (the medical lead[17]) and a champion (the medical director[18] at the time). The medical director took the lead in accessing resources (a room, lunches, publicity, and communications support) and encouraging staff at all levels of the organisation to support this new intervention. In this way he took the pressure from the facilitators who then could focus on finding stories and telling them safely. These staff whose support the medical lead enlisted included the chief executive and the chair, a steering group of managers and clinicians, senior and junior staff, and, importantly, both converts and cynics.

The early steering group meetings were in essence a microcosm of the process to come, as stories and speakers were considered and the purpose and process of the Round misunderstood and clarified. Each misunderstanding deepened the thinking of the Rounds champions, who through the process became clearer about how to position Rounds. In managing the early challenges, the future shape of the Rounds began to form, and the processes within them and underpinning them began to be conceptualised.

In essence these meetings were the first place where the anxiety about creating a non–hierarchical, organisation-wide forum, in which the purpose was reflection not action, was acted out. To clear a whole hour of work time, and within it to sanction not acting or reacting was countercultural. There was immense early pressure to identify ways to "capture the learning" or to put in place systems to support those "who might be upset" by a Round. The lack of confidence in the ability of the organisation

---

[17]Dr Mark Harber, consultant in renal medicine.
[18]Dr Adrian Tookman, consultant in palliative medicine, now clinical director, Marie Curie.

to publicly witness the pain, cost, and rewards of the work without "taking action" was striking. Throughout the organisation on a daily basis, staff members were being buffeted by the fallout from the intense emotional experiences which patients (and their families) were experiencing, and exposed to trauma and loss and high stress often with extreme organisational ambivalence about what support might be warranted. Now with the prospect of creating a monthly neutral space within which *anything* could be said, or experienced, or noticed by *anyone*, there was a low-level panic.

It needed the psychologist to resist the proposal to promote psychology services at the Schwartz Round before kneejerk reactions to the worry about an unmanageable emotional reaction to the Rounds could be managed. It seemed vital to challenge these worries, which, though an understandable expression of anxiety (as organisational defences are powerful and necessary), would result in a splitting in the positioning of the Rounds. That is, there was a risk was that they would be seen as a forum for "discussing feelings" rather than an opportunity to bear witness to many varieties of clinical and organisational experience. Within this risk was the possibility that they could be diluted and devalued by being consigned to being a space for "soft" talk rather than for the exploration of the qualities, resources, and courage required to work with hard realities. In this reflex action to the anxiety they raised (expressed most commonly as the need to look after staff who might be traumatised by a Round) there was much potential for both minimising and pathologising emotional experience through, amongst other things, the implication that realistic emotional distress requires professional intervention.

So an initial conceptualisation of the Round was required in response. In fact it soon became clear that each challenge in implementing Rounds was an expression of one (mis)understanding of emotional experience (and of the process of intervention to manage it) and that the best response to these challenges was to suggest a different understanding. In this case, for example, it seemed that some people might be viewing a Schwartz Round as some kind of intense psychotherapeutic process which ran the risk of leaving attenders undefended and unable to cope, or to return to work, after their one hour's experience.

The organisation was encouraged instead to consider a Round as a community intervention acting in the context of a network of relationships within which there were resources that could be mobilised both within, but importantly also outside, the Round, to enable attenders to manage the impact of the stories. In fact the deepening of relationships, which this process implies, may be one of the benefits of a Schwartz Round. It was suggested that perhaps over time the process of not reacting to the worry about whether the emotional reality of health-care work could be publicly named and withstood would build individual and organisational confidence. It might increase the ability to pay attention to and manage both inner and private experiences without the fear of abandonment, or of being emotionally overwhelmed, or criticised by self or others, or of provoking some form of retaliation.

This process also suggested the value of paying attention to language and the management of paradox already described in Part II, in positioning the Rounds. Though they are an intervention whose success is dependent on psychological thinking and understanding, it seemed very important in the early stages to ally them with non–psychological language and with other professional groups. The aim of integration of experience (personal with professional, for example) that is at the heart of this intervention needed to be mirrored in the process of implementation. Bringing together different areas of the hospital would make it more likely that they would become connected to all strands of organisational life. In this way the hope was that they would bring forth stories that would be of relevance to staff who would never naturally ally themselves to psychology, or feelings, or reflective space. Or to soft talk—though the psychology service had already borne witness to the fact that it is the soft stuff that is the toughest to manage, and shapes the relationship to work and to organisational life and perhaps to patients.

The search for a first story

With the infrastructure in place and an emerging understanding of a Round developing, the work now turned to planning and preparing the first Round. Where would we start? Which panel would go first? Through discussion in the steering group a recent case was chosen. It was known to staff on the steering group who was troubled by the memory of the distress that staff had experienced due to the inability of a family to accept a diagnosis and treatment plan for a relative. A father who was a patient on one of the wards had been seriously ill and had needed high levels of pain medication. The dose needed to keep him comfortable also made him sleepy. His family, sensing correctly that he was slipping away from them, did not want him to be medicated to a level when he could no longer speak much or be available to them and were pressurising the medical team to lower the medication dose. In the middle was the nursing team, witnessing the distress that this disagreement was causing the man, especially at night when he was alone and neither his family nor the prescribing medical team were available.

The case was chosen because it would provide an opportunity to reflect on many themes of relevance to clinicians. It was called "Caught between the patient and their family", which suggested the not uncommon experience of feeling unable to get it right for everyone in a family and the accompanying fear that in this process the patient could slip out of view. It also raised a consideration, which was to surface in many a future Round, which was the question of just who is the patient in a complex case? Who takes up the team's energy? The awareness of how the focus of clinical work can be diverted because of one family member's emotional needs also allowed for an expression of another concern that was to be explored in different ways in many future Rounds: the worry that those who shout loudest get more.

The varying experience of staff due to their relative presence or absence, for example a medical consultant's guilty awareness of making decisions that nursing staff are then left to implement and deal with the fallout from, were also present in this Round. As was the anger that has to be suppressed by clinicians when they watch a family attempt to pressure them in a way that will cause pain to their patient. Suppressed in order to hopefully help the family realise the reality of their situation and the impact of their poor choice. All these themes emerged in the Round, as did the riskier topic of the feelings that need to be managed when working with a family whom you don't like.

The first Round

All through the journey from the UK to the US and back we had carried one question with us. Would Schwartz Rounds translate to the UK? Would healthcare staff in London open up and use them? Would anybody come? But when we ran this first Round we were overwhelmed by the numbers as ninety staff attended, and it felt immediately as if we were tapping into a strong need. We were surprised at how eagerly the space was immediately used and then, when one of the clinicians in the audience responded to the themes above by saying that it was not the families that she didn't like who worried her but those for whom she could feel little, we knew we were onto something important.

From that moment we felt instinctively that when provided with stories which created permission for unspoken fears to be surfaced, people would use this space to discuss risky and authentic experiences they were exposed to in their relationships with patients and families, because of their deep need to try to help and cure. One authentic risky statement (about the fear of feeling little, which was balanced in many later Rounds by a consideration of the opposite experience: the difficulty of managing the intensity of the emotional aspects of healthcare work) gave us the conviction to continue. As did the fact that though we, the facilitators, had worried about how we would manage silence in such a large group, in the event our main task became how to channel, manage, and properly close the flow of words and emotion that emerged in response to this poignant story. Looking back on that first Round we realised that a story had been offered that had allowed us to craft an opportunity for staff to express how they grappled with the emotional complexity and the multiple contexts of their work. We were on our way, and maybe only subconsciously appreciated that we would now need to balance a search for stories with allowing the emerging themes to shape *us*, as we tried to steady ourselves in this risky, uncertain, and exposing business of facilitating the unknown quantity which at that time a Schwartz Round in the UK was. The various elements of this process will now be described.

Story catching and some food for thought

Over the months that followed we sought out and were offered stories to be told at the Rounds. In these early Rounds we chose carefully to ensure the speakers would be able to confidently and safely tell a good story in front of a large group (we were getting over 100 people attending each Round) in a way that connected their personal and professional selves in the storytelling. We chose stories that moved or inspired us and that we felt would give permission for attenders to respond with stories of their own. We hoped that they would surface experiences that up until now had only been heard by the psychologist, and even then often brought to her with a wish to leave them discreetly behind in her office forever. Now there was a chance to reverse the direction of travel, to bring these experiences centre stage in the hope that they could become a meal to be digested in public, rather than a worrying shadow to be split off and abandoned.

At the end of each Round, we invited people to offer us stories for future Rounds and the offerings we received told us much about the current preoccupations of staff within their clinical work and in terms of organisational life. Through this process we got to meet many new people in the organisation and hear about the widely varied work they did, what they were worried about, what they were proud of, exhausted from, what saddened and puzzled, infuriated and frightened, humbled and inspired them.

Being a facilitator gave us permission to follow the flow of stories that swirled around the hospital and became a legitimate way to connect to the many tributaries from these stories that trickled away into all of its far corners. To quiet, silent places, where patients were held safe and tenderly cared for by staff under huge pressure. To noisy, busy wards where terrible losses were borne and tough decisions made, while clinics were kept running and fresh beds were made for the next batch of patients: to theatres where technology and humans kept watch over sleeping patients while cutting and repairing them; to many other wards and clinics where hopeful, joyful, and funny moments were celebrated; and to offices and corridors where loneliness and conflict, fear and personal needs were silenced and suppressed, in order that the work of the hospital could continue to be done.

We followed the ripples that flowed out from the stories told at each Round and traced the new seams that were revealed, and they brought us to all of these and many more places, and to a deeper understanding of organisational life in all its messy complexity. We brought back with us stories that needed to be told, and we used the impact which they had had on us to consider how best to tell them, in order that they could be truly and constructively heard.

We would be offered "topics" for future Rounds and in terms of content this is what they were. Somebody would say: "We think it might be good to do a Round on organ retrieval. Would you like to hear our story?" But when we travelled out to hear them what we were often met with was a hope for containment and an unspoken wish for help with processing the complex meaning of the individual and team experience that underpinned the story, as well as a desire to go public with the work for a variety of reasons. Being a psychologist deepened the preparation work, informing the story catching, the thinking about the purpose of the storytelling, and the growing belief that to do this work effectively and safely the storytellers must be properly prepared.

Crafting stories and co-creating meaning: panel preparation

Looking back, the decision to spend time preparing the panel emerged from the experience of providing the psychology services. This work had shown how much staff underestimated the emotional impact of their work, which left unacknowledged could then emerge in unconscious expressions of emotional distress: a team scapegoating one of its members, for example, rather than addressing the helplessness engendered by the work, or a distance developing in relationships with patients being used, as an unconscious strategy to manage the impact of limited resources. It had also demonstrated the value of exploring the personal and professional meaning of work experiences, and the power of both the telling of a story and of being heard.

In our meetings with the first panels we heard striking, powerful, humbling, and moving stories. Sometimes we watched the storytellers weep, or try not to weep, as they revisited their experiences. We were in awe of the work they did and what they managed to achieve as well as what they had to withstand in this work. We were struck (and sometimes surprised) by the eagerness of many panellists to tell their story in public but aware of our responsibility to them to ensure that it was a safe, productive experience for them. The urge to confess seemed sometimes to override the need to pay attention to the rules of organisational life.

Despite all these multiple and in some cases conflicting layers of possibility in relation to each story which we were offered, we could, however, sense the potential to help panellists to attend to their stories in a way that would reveal the personal meaning that had underpinned their emotional experience of this work (conscious or unconscious though it may have been at the time). We worked with the panellists to help them to then craft the stories so that they were organised simply and solely around this meaning in order to benefit both the storyteller and the listening group. We aimed to open spaces for new stories to emerge (Freedman & Coombs, 1996).

We could sense the potential for public storytelling to be a healing and therapeutic experience. But we were also aware of our responsibility to the audience, many of whom would be as affected as we were by what they heard. However, anticipating the emotional reaction of the audience helped shape our approach to the storytelling for surely here there was a chance to create resonance in a way that would be productive for the group and could allow for the safe release of emotion.

If an individual experience became linked to universal themes and this link could emerge in the crafting of the story, then perhaps personal exposure could become an opportunity for group witnessing rather than for isolation and judgement. We knew of course that though the position we were taking as listeners and facilitators who were helping panellists to tell (and then to craft) their stories was one of neutral curiosity that the context in which the stories were to be told was not neutral. It was a hierarchical, rule bound, competitive, and occasionally unforgiving context.

For the storyteller, the panel preparation provided an opportunity to consider the impact of the experience of their work in relation to its emotional significance. Why had this case felt difficult, rewarding, enriching, frustrating, or impossible? What was most significant—the content of the work, the people involved, the team and organisational support, the relationship between this case and their own personal story, etc.? What factors had made it easier or more difficult for the work to be done? What strategies had they used to cope with the challenges posed by the case (clinical, organisational) and manage their own internal experiences at the same time? Why had they decided to offer this story (amongst all the many stories they could tell) for a Schwartz Round? What might this be telling us about them, their team, their speciality, this organisation, and the UK healthcare context right now? Through the process of telling and retelling, multiple layers of context emerged.[19]

Storytelling without means or ends

Asking systemically informed questions, teasing out the impact of layers of meaning, and focussing on the personal experience within a professional role, all provided a new lens within which the panellists could observe and consider the stories which they brought. In this way the stories began to take shape, and the space between the story and the storyteller began to emerge. Within this space the relationship to work and to organisational life could be discerned and the neutral observation of experience slowly became possible. We aimed to help panellists see themselves from a new position and to move them from

---

[19]See Wren (2013) for a further discussion of systemic and narrative techniques in panel preparation.

the landscape of action (the sequence of events) to the landscape of identity (the needs, drives, values, beliefs, commitments that underpinned action) (Bruner, 1986; White, 2014). And we also planned to mirror this process in the facilitation of the Round—to create a space in which observation without action was possible. Within this space, where the undertow of experience was suggested, implicit values, conscious and unconscious drives, organisational imperatives, political realities, and personal histories would slowly become discernible. Ultimately these layers of experience could be used to craft stories in the preparation of the panel, and to develop themes and positions in the facilitation of the Round.

Early on we realised that storytellers would often try to help us organise the stories they told us around an action—learning for example, or reflection, or review—common activities associated with storytelling in learning organisations. In this way they were conveying an implicit assumption about activity that was valued in this context, and also an expectation of what we sought. That is evidence of improvement, of learning, of *productivity* essentially, non-productive activity not being sanctioned in healthcare organisations. Thus the stories, though often emerging in a chaotic, unformed, and emotionally fraught way would often be forced by the storyteller towards a point of learning or achievement, for this was the context within which experience was typically explored—with an end in mind. So within the storytelling a process of assessment and of judgement was being implicitly adhered to. For example, we would be told about what an individual and/or team had gained or learned from a difficult experience, what they wished they had done differently, or what they were proud of in the work. These evaluations were the frames that were offered to us to hold the experiences the storytellers wished to bring to the Round.

But we resisted this because we were striving to move from the realm of productivity to the realm of aesthetics (Pearce, 1976) and the creation of meaning. In this realm we aimed to open a space within which there was no requirement to be productive, the pressures created by conscious and unconscious organisational, professional, or personal imperatives could be noticed, and the relief in temporarily relinquishing them could simply be experienced. We aimed to temporarily separate the person from the role, the act from the responsibility to act, the work from the organisational rules that governed it, and ultimately "the dancer from the dance".

Repositioning: self and story

And so the panel preparation resisted the frames of reference and the direction of travel, which we were implicitly offered, and simply stayed curious about how the interaction between personal, professional, team, and organisational contexts had informed the emotional experience that occurred in relation to this piece of work. We worked to stay empathetically interested in how this experience had developed and to truly understand its impact. We helped craft the stories by staying close and true to emerging themes, the fault lines of personal, clinical, and organisational life in healthcare. And we used our response to the stories to feedback possibilities of meaning, drawing on systemic and psychodynamic theory both to make sense of emerging understanding and to contain the process.

This created the possibility for the authentic storytelling, which is at the heart of successful Rounds and enables the group to move towards the emotion within each story. In this way they are both temporarily released from rules of this hierarchical setting, able to respond to the simple humanity of the storyteller (regardless of role), and also given permission to connect freely to similar emotional experiences of their own. It is the panel preparation that enables this key process to occur and allows the Round to achieve the goal of a communal witnessing of staff experience. It also overcomes some of the risks of this large group activity, most significantly the risk of breaching any patient confidentiality because the focus of the storytelling has shifted away from the patient even before the Round has begun.

Repositioning: team and story

As well as repositioning the storytellers in relation to their story this preparation process also repositions the panellists in relation to each other. Usually a panel is made up of members of a team all discussing a case on which they had worked. Panel preparation meetings allow them to hear more about the real impact of a case on other members of the team. It also often revealed interactions between a patient and/or family members that other team members hadn't been aware of and thus created a new understanding of the work and of relationships within the team. By staying curious about the team's experience (rather than the patients'—where the realm of productivity is active and the imperative towards diagnosis, prognosis, treatment, and quick discharge leads to a form of shorthand being used to speed up, prioritise, and get through a story as quickly as possible), new details can emerge along with a new understanding of how the range of (known and unknown, shared and withheld) individual experiences combine to create the team's relationship to the treatment of a patient and his family.

Discussing a case from this new position allows for new possibilities of connection and relationship to the work to emerge. It also creates a feeling of space and time to attend to details that might not seem obviously relevant. Though in the great scheme of things they are very brief, these moments of paying attention to staff experience work in the opposite direction to organisational life where behaviour is more and more often based on the common belief that there is *no* space and *no* time, especially for staff needs. Simply reversing this process for a panel preparation meeting aims to suggest a new possibility, a different way of paying attention. The deepening of understanding that tends to emerge becomes its own reward and the value of reflection is experienced. Any resultant shift in thinking and connection occurs through the often unexpected emotional experience of the storytelling that is encouraged, and the subsequent repositioning. The crafting of the story connects the emotional experience to the cognitive, the patient's story to the clinician's story, the personal to the professional experience, and individuals to the team.

Hearing yourself think

Speaking the story out loud is key and from quite early on the benefit of getting the panellists in the preparation meeting to just tell the story for five minutes, one after the other, without interruption, became apparent. This overcame the tendency for staff to "say what they were going to say", refer to patient notes, check background details, make sure they remembered it right, etc. Instead it allowed each of them, and their colleagues, to try to tell a story by seeing and hearing what filled the five minute space first, and to notice the impact of the stories on each other. The subsequent discussion and reaction began the process of unravelling the stories and teasing out the unique individual experiences and the common themes. If there was time a second meeting would then be held when panellists would bring their now more developed stories to rehearse, having established a key focus and gained a clearer sense of how their experience related to that of the rest of the team. The order of the stories and the anticipation of the experience of public storytelling could then be discussed and planned for.

The shift in the focus of interest from the patient to the storyteller that is the central pivot of a panel preparation meeting acts as a real but also a symbolic expression of interest in staff experience. It is interesting to reflect on the cumulative cultural impact of this repetitive expression of interest and curiosity about individual experience within which it is hoped that the following sentiment is being expressed by the preparer of the panel to the storyteller ...

"Your experience matters to, and interests me (the organisationally sanctioned listener to stories, with no brief to act on them beyond ensuring that they are heard). Tell me (again and again and again) why it matters to you. Help me help you to shape it. And I will think about what I hear and use both my emotional and professional response to plan and facilitate a Round in which your experience is both amplified—through the creation of resonance, and personalised—through the excavation and exploration of authenticity, in order for the group to consider and better understand the uniqueness of your individual experience in the context of the universality of the themes and issues dealt with in healthcare work."

And so this rolling wave of meaning pulls like the tide towards itself in each single movement (reflecting a unique individual experience) but is also continually being pulled back to a greater shared space within which there are many undercurrents, rough waters, clashing drifts, and huge swells; and further out an immense deep, silent, and wordless expanse within which our common humanity can be temporarily held safe, witnessed, and acknowledged. Put simply, the aim of the panel preparation is to move away from activity and productivity, and towards stillness, silence, and observation, by facilitating the telling of stories that can suggest many true experiences that often feel beyond words—both for our patients and for ourselves.

Repositioning: the prospect of now being heard

Panel preparation then is a process of helping panellists to tell their stories in order to create meaning and to reposition them in the first instance in relation to their experience. It also aims to get the optimal balance between the revisiting of experience and the anticipation of the future public storytelling, and in this way to reposition the storytellers again, but this time in relation to their organisational context. Thus the second part of this process aims to create a holding framework within which panellists can not only connect with the emotional impact of their story, but also with the anticipated emotion associated with telling it in public. We worked to manage the subtle complexities involved in this process and get the safest balance between (sometimes new or emerging) self and team awareness, and future public exposure. Occasionally we would decide to postpone a Round because the time was not right to achieve this balance, the experience was too recent, emotion was too raw, or the preparation revealed team issues or organisational issues that needed to be addressed before a story could safely be told.

Balancing the intimacy of storytelling with a public performance

In anticipating the experience of public storytelling, panellists were able to express and discuss their associated anxieties. While the starting point was often the common experience of fear of public speaking, further exploration would allow for a consideration of the spoken and unspoken rules about what aspects of experience could be publicly acknowledged and discussed, or expressed as a fear of being overwhelmed by emotion, or of being judged or criticised, or of confidentiality being breached for example. Another common and interesting anxiety was that an experience was not important or significant enough to warrant sharing it in a public forum. The panel preparation process provided an opportunity to resist this common tendency to minimise personal experience. Often the distinction between a performance (such as an impressive presentation) and a simple authentic story would need to be discussed with panellists, because of course it was the simple authentic stories that had the most power. Junior staff may have been more likely to worry about whether an experience was important enough to warrant this attention. Senior staff understandably often struggled to drop their professional persona. The more that difficult experiences could be understood and discussed in the preparation, the greater the permission we would subsequently obtain to introduce them as themes for consideration in the Round. For example, how risky is it for a senior staff member to discuss doubt, despair, and fear? Can she resume her role afterwards? What is it like to worry that you might be making too much of a painful experience that you can't seem to shake off? Who decides what experiences are worth paying attention to and how do they decide? Of course, simply telling stories on the panel within which these dilemmas were obvious had great power to give permission for members of the group to reconsider their attitude to these very questions.

Ruptures, safety, and opportunity

What we were ultimately discussing in this process of creating safe passage for individual experiences was how we could manage the ruptures involved in bringing a private experience into a public forum in a way that would ensure that no important professional authority could be permanently lost in the cracks which these ruptures could possibly open up. In fact the cracks, the fault lines, were the spaces we wanted to create in order to suggest the universal difficulties of integration, the need for flexibility, the benefits of self-compassion, the impossibility sometimes of staying in touch with feelings when at work, and the potential time lag between an event and its impact.

The pressure to effectively manage these potential ruptures is a key part of facilitator anxiety when beginning Rounds, but when well-prepared, good Rounds allow these cracks to become evident, considered, and discussed, and the process usually leads to a deepening of professional authority in, and of respect for, the storyteller. The development of an understanding of the connection between the hurt that can be caused by the work, and the courage required to withstand and discuss it, becomes possible. The connection between the pain and the development of creativity becomes evident. The emergence of compassion becomes inevitable and irresistible.

In this process of anticipating the performance and its risks, the stories were shaped, their central significance further understood, and decisions were then made about what would be the main focus when the time came to tell the story in the Round in a five minute slot. The short time available created a pressure for a focussed story, made the organisation of meaning tighter, and now pulled the storyteller towards the performance requirement of the Round. Moving from exploration, which had widened the lens of the storytelling to now planning to perform, created a pressure in which the unpacked story was reorganised around one or two focal points. The storyteller was reassured that the facilitator would also hold the memory of the story from preparation and could amplify and deepen themes and introduce elements that had been forgotten. In this way the storyteller was left with the responsibility of managing time and staying authentic, but was reassured that the facilitator would take responsibility for the process, including what was not said but remembered, what was evoked, and what might be avoided within the Round.

While this preparation process also concerned the aesthetics of the Round, ensuring that for the audience the performance aspect had cohesion and coherence, it also positioned the facilitator as holding the responsibility for ensuring that the link between private experience and public knowledge was managed safely and sensitively. In this way the facilitator role mirrored the role of the psychologist already described, in its movement from the private to the public experience and back again. In this movement there was the symbolic possibility of making the boundaries between these two arenas of experience become both more permeable and paradoxically more obvious, and to instil confidence in the ability to flexibly manage transitions between the two.

Facilitating: creating resonance, amplifying authenticity, and the power of suggestion

With the preparation done the Round can be begin. The facilitators place themselves at the boundary between public and private experience at the very beginning of the Round by visibly drawing a line around the one-hour space. They describe what it will be like, how it will begin and end, how it is different from the other hours of the day in this organisation. They tell the group how they wish them to treat the stories that they will hear and how it is hoped the relationship to experience will be explored once the stories have been told and invite them to share any memories and feelings that are evoked by them. The panellists then speak and tell their stories one by one without interruption.

The speaking gives permission for private stories to now be heard in public places, for individuals to listen and as they listen to consider the personal resources and values they draw on to do their work. There is permission for stories of creativity, hope, tenderness, shame, guilt, love, fear, anger, and regret to emerge in a group setting. This performance of the stories usually has a powerful impact on both the storytellers and the listeners, palpable in the quality of the listening and in the fullness of the silences. The opportunity to be inspired and moved, the chance to feel part of a community and not alone, the glimpses of aspects of personal and organisational life that once were hidden, and the group witnessing of experience are all part of this initial, silent, and often very moving impact.

From the story to the group

Once they are finished the facilitators open out to the group for their reaction and response. In the early Rounds this proved to be the most anxiety-provoking phase for us. We worried about silence, we were anxious about what could and should come next. We were also employees of the organisation, influenced by its culture and bound by its rules. How much permission would it give us, or could we seize, to create a neutral space in which observation and experience without action was possible and permissible?

Over time we learned to hold the silence more confidently, to begin to develop our own authority, and to grow surer of our ability to resist the pull towards action. We drew some of this authority from the huge and immediate endorsement of the process which we received from staff both within and outside the Round. We also came to understand that silences were a reflection of uncertainty about how to engage with this new space. They would often be paralleled by a pull towards problem solving or to rescuing the participants. The urge to tidy, repair, and make better was strong and hard to resist. We knew that it was important to try to model how to use a Round by creating thoughtful, confident, and paced movements in the facilitation, drawing on the themes that had emerged in the preparation as we steadied ourselves in order to move confidently through the silent, full spaces, and the busy, distracting, work-like ones. By resisting the problem solving, though often noticing it and naming it, by considering aloud the impact of the implicit sense of rules that may have prompted it, the facilitation could slowly nudge the group towards a position of curiosity about experiences, those of the storytellers and their own. This tussle between the old and the new use of "empty" spaces, that is, between production and digestion, would usually take up at least the first half of the Round.

But if (and we weren't always successful) the facilitation had managed to keep returning to a position of neutral curiosity, then in the second half a different process, that of resonance (Carey & Russell,

2013), would emerge. The group would begin to share memory and experience as if thinking aloud. They would become freer to name and explore experiences that mirrored the panel stories, the themes would become naturally amplified and deepened, and the many layers of context would begin to emerge. Facilitation could thicken this process by moving to and from micro and macro level experience, by considering both the uniqueness of a story and the universality of the experience. It could explore issues of power, control, fear, and flexibility; and themes of loss, hope, joy, creativity, and generativity (and their opposites) that were at the heart of the stories, just as they sit at the centre of every important life experience. While attending to individual experience in order to explore meaning, the facilitation could suggest the widest canvas on which this meaning could be considered, as befitted the context of initial stories and the time available. The awareness of time, the need to finish promptly and to resist the urge to tidy up as we finished, all informed the process of the second half and of the closing of a Round. In our minds we knew that in a month's time we would open the space for an hour again.

Our initial aim was to provide digestible food for thought in a paced and contained way, different enough but not so different that the experience would be rejected. Over time, through the support we received for the process, through attendance, engagement, and offers of stories, we knew we could go further with the use of this space. But in the beginning we simply wanted to suggest possibilities, and to convey a sense that we could discern needs and anticipate fears and translate them into productive storytelling. We wanted to develop the group's confidence that the shape of the stories that would be told could in some part match the shape of the experiences they were carrying inside their bodies and their minds, carried in some cases in words and stories and in others cases in a place beyond language and expression.

Here are seven of the stories.

PART IV

Seven true tales

Resetting and restoring
A punch in the stomach, a blink in the eye

Just as some stories are more powerful than others, some Rounds seem
to pack more of a punch—
it isn't just that the stories themselves are powerful—
though they are—
It's that they surprise you—
the whole thing surprises you and leaves you wondering but what
was that?—(I thought I was just having a normal day at work)
at the same time you know it was something unique, something
unrepeatable and special, only of that moment and place in time
when you had a glimpse of something deeply intimate and private,
and yet familiar—
and closer maybe to a diary or a play or poem or than to "work"—
but the power of course is that it's real and not "pretend"—
yet making the **art of work** momentarily visible.

As well as the movement of the storytelling in the
room there is stillness
and in the stillness a deep respect for the storyteller, and for the shape
of his story which seems to convey something about the shape of the
world inside him, and the shape of the family he came from, and the
families he is making with his work ...

And every organisation has a Round that lodges
itself deep in memory—
not abstract memory but memory as a fibrous textured
space that you could run your fingers along

—Meshed together with sinews, and muscle and bone—
—and fragments of heart and blood
—memory that speaks and says—**this is who we are,**
this is what we do—memory that crafts identity
—at the same time as creating a desire for identity
—and carries the hope—
—(just for a moment)—

of belonging to an inspirational tribe

Tripped up by a teddy: a surgeon's tale

Some Rounds seem pivotal, deepening the organisation's understanding of their power, moving the space towards new depths. They showcase the complexity of clinical work, its impact, and the graceful way it is managed. They lodge themselves deep in the organisation's memory.

This first tale is of one example of this: an early Round with a panel of four members of the transplant team. Some panellists did the organ retrieval only. Others did organ retrieval and transplantation. They got to see both sides of the story: the losses and the gains. Each panellist described one incident he had experienced in this work. The surgeon's story took place when he was a senior registrar, new to leading the team, feeling confident about being a surgeon, keen to teach junior doctors and to demonstrate his skills. He described having a patient who needed a transplant and getting a call to say there was an organ available. He travelled to another hospital to collect it; full of confidence, aware of the happy anticipation of the expectant, hopeful patient in the hospital he would return to. At the time he said he felt like a strong macho doctor, enjoying leading his team, ready to demonstrate his skill and authority.

As the retrieval surgery ended and the surgical drapes were removed from the donor he noticed a rustle of paper below the body of the child donating the organs and then something fell on the floor. It was a teddy bear. The mother knowing that her child, the donor, would die once the retrieval was over, wanted the teddy the child had been given on the day he was born to be with him for this, the last hours of his life. The rustle of paper were some pages on which the child's family had made the imprint of their hands so that he would die in their arms. Once the transplant co-ordinator explained this to the surgeon he described how the "ring of steel around his emotions was broken" and he had to leave the room to gather himself. The full implication of what he was doing flooded through him. He realised he had been so caught up with the good he was doing for the recipient family and filled with a sense of his skill and power at this stage of his career, that he had had little time to consider the implications of the retrieval process for the donor family. In the panel preparation session he had wept when he told this part of the story and we had discussed with him how he would like to manage this in the Schwartz Round. We were all new to Rounds, we all shared some anxiety about a senior consultant crying in public, and we didn't want it to be a negative experience for him. As facilitators we also wondered how we would feel and manage. It was a very moving story to hear. We advised him to leave out any part of the story that felt too difficult to tell on the day. Perhaps he could describe the impact of the experience without mentioning the teddy, which seemed to be the trigger for the tears each time we rehearsed the story.

I remember arriving at the Round and placing a packet of tissues on the table because I had a cold and the surgeon thanked me for bringing them. We joked about who the tissues were for but again we advised him to relate only what he was comfortable with. However, as soon as he started the story it was obvious that he was headed straight for the detail of the teddy. That was the first thing I remember about that Round, the way he gathered up all his energy and went straight to the heart of the story, revealing a very moving and true personal experience within a professional role. The second thing was the complete silence in the room as he spoke. The stillness spoke not just of the level of emotion but also of the respect with which his story was being received, and perhaps an element of surprise to get this type of insight into a surgeon's experience.

There were two other details that stayed with me. The surgeons on the panel who did retrievals described how they always finished by writing "Thank you" in the medical notes, because they know that this will be the last ever entry in the notes. This seemed like such a sensitive and thoughtful gesture to me, so respectful of the generosity that was taking place amid huge loss. It was very moving. I remember wondering if patients and families know that they do that? Do they realise with how much care and thought their sadness is handled? Or how much healthcare professionals are affected by and mindful of the losses of their patients and their families. The second detail was that as the surgeon was finishing his teddy story he looked up to a man who had just arrived and was sitting down at the back of the room and said, "Hi Dad." His father, the surgeon responsible for setting up the whole transplant service had arrived to hear his son's story.

It was a very poignant Round that everyone who attended remembers and it continues to be talked about. Afterwards the surgeon told me that it was the first time he had ever told the teddy story without crying. The room itself felt full of tears: of the images of the teddy; the handprints; the quiet, sensitive "Thank you's" in the notes; a sense that there was a family right here in the room—a son performing for his father who had given him the love of this work in the first place—and an audience slightly stunned but completely gratified to hear this compelling story of important but complex work and the profound emotions behind it. The power of a Schwartz Round to reveal delicate and surprising connections between the personal and the professional and to demonstrate the thought, care, and emotional investment of health professionals was palpable. As was one of the truths that seemed to emerge from the stories and the subsequent discussion:

In healthcare, as in life, to get on with the business of living we must let go of the dead. But it is a wrench and we must find ways to acknowledge our guilt at living and our grief or we will become unable to act. The Round seemed to capture the literal knife edge along which healthcare work moves, poised between life and death, needing to find the right spaces to acknowledge both when appropriate, and to block them out too when needed. The potential for Rounds to integrate experiences that need to be fragmented in order for the work to take place was starting to become apparent.

Why don't you go back where you came from?
Tales of hurt and anger

One of the topics regularly returned to in Schwartz Rounds is of bad behaviour towards staff, either by a patient or by a family member. This can range from mildly upsetting and annoying to very toxic and aversive behaviour, which may lead to security guards, professional bodies, or in some case the police needing to be involved. Once a story is unpacked, what lies beneath, unsurprisingly, is often a very damaged or distressed personality, or a complex family dynamic. In relation to Schwartz Rounds what is important is not this analysis, but the impact on staff and the reality of what they have to withstand.

One Schwartz Round was about staff experience of dealing with such a personality, a woman using renal services over an extended period of time. This is a context with its own emotional complexities where because of the need for dialysis there is often a long-standing dependent relationship between patient and staff. The overt reliance of the patient on the ongoing treatment forces both patients and staff into a type of unremitting intimacy within which complex emotions need to be managed. Occasionally, self-destructive behaviour can emerge which can be very difficult for healthcare staff to witness. These panellists' stories in this Round highlighted how this woman coped with the experience of extreme stress by alienating those around her. In the panel preparation sessions we discussed how the greater her need, the more damage she did to the opportunities the healthcare team offered her for comfort and kindness, for some solace and reassurance. It seemed as if she was expressing her deep rage at the loss of control her illness was wreaking on her by inflicting a negative control on the staff that were caring for her. By inflicting pain she could guarantee that they would be stretched to the limits of their compassion and tolerance. Maybe she could transmit to them some of the experience of the revulsion she was having at the way her body was letting her down. Because she knew that they knew that her life depended on them she would try to force them to tolerate completely unacceptable and abusive behaviour. Would they dare to reject her? Might one of them lose control and let herself down in the way she was feeling let down? She was a patient of the service over a number of years and the team saw her social circumstances change and her disease become more serious and bleak. Despite her behaviour towards them it was clear that they were able to maintain compassion until the end perhaps because of the sadness of her plight.

There are two things I remember about this Round. One was the extent of the vicious behaviour that staff had to withstand from this woman. At one stage of the woman's treatment the senior nurse on the panel was pregnant and the patient said she hoped that the baby in her womb would die. When she told this story on the panel there was a ripple of horror through the room. The other thing I remember was the dignity and creativity in the way staff withstood the attacks on them. Another nurse on the panel, who was black, told how the patient would say to him, "Why don't you go back to where you came from? … What are you doing here anyway?" and he would drop, rather than raise his voice and tell her quietly that he was here because he had travelled a long way and trained specially to learn how to look after people like her. He had a stillness and a quiet presence about him in his storytelling that seemed to hint at a wise flexibility and a resilience that enabled him to reach deep into his own humanity rather than react negatively in the face of such provocation. Both members of staff though tempted to withdraw from the patient managed somehow to do the opposite.

When the subject of bullying, harassment, or racism comes up at Schwartz Rounds someone will inevitably say, "But don't we have a policy for this kind of unacceptable behaviour?" In this Round someone in the audience asked the black nurse—"But didn't that make you angry?" And both questions seem in some ways superfluous. Because of course this behaviour makes people justifiably very angry; yes, there are policies and of course there is zero tolerance for this kind of behaviour but that does not remove the necessity to experience it sometimes and to have to choose a response, in the moment, to provocation. Nor does it change the fact that the people behaving this badly are desperately ill and vulnerable. When this is raised in the Round, immediately and rightly someone will point out that other people are desperately ill and don't behave like that. "My need or yours?" is the stark equation that begins to emerge in discussions in such Rounds. Various versions of "Staff have needs and rights too" are expressed, which leads to the next thought, that "There has to be a limit to what we are asked to do." The thought that comes after that is of course: *there has to be a limit to our compassion.* But who will dare say this and who will decide what that is and how we set the limit?

Often in Rounds like this it feels like we are tiptoeing on taboos, or that eggshells of implicit rules and values are being smashed, or maybe just crunched gently underfoot as social problems and psychiatric presentations stretch healthcare workers to full capacity and make them question the balance between what is being required of them, what they have left to give, and the containment and support they are being offered, while they withstand bad behaviour. And in the storytelling it usually becomes clear that it is individual resources (values, humour, spirituality, flexibility, personal experience, fondness for patients and their families, an ability to withstand the mad chaos, commitment to the NHS) and local team support that enable staff to withstand experiences like this.

Patients like these breach the invisible contract that enables staff to stay close to aversive and unpleasant experience. The contract states that a) patients' needs are greater than ours and b) patients are usually dependent and largely grateful. That is, the power dynamic is clear and its rules make the transactions in the healthcare relationship manageable. Once the contract is breached, we become overly aware of our own needs and the patient destroys our goodwill through destructive ingratitude; then the need to reject the patient and protect ourselves is unleashed. The special rules of healthcare (invested in individuals and held safe by organisational and professional structures), which make possible the intimacy with strangers that underpins the work, are disbanded.

Rounds can provide a safe space for a consideration of this unpleasant experience. They create an opportunity to imagine this intimate relationship without boundaries. They provide permission for discussion of forbidden impulses that violate our view of ourselves, for example: the desire to retaliate against a patient, the need sometimes to manage extreme dislike or detachment, or to acknowledge anger, and feelings of violence towards patients, and their families. To name these feelings is to reduce their power over us and Rounds like this provide opportunities for profound relief and normalisation. How much better a group acknowledgement of this unboundaried experience than a referral to psychology to consider in private those unmentionable feelings that we imagine "nobody else has". Through reflection and consideration, through an acknowledgement that this experience of aggression is a problem for this hospital community (because of doing healthcare work in this society right now), the unmentionable is mentioned, a sense of isolation is reduced, and the risk of unmanageable feelings taking hold and being acted on is hopefully reduced. And junior staff are privy to the thoughts, feelings, and coping strategies of senior consultants and senior nurses to which they would not normally have access and vice versa. Rounds provide an opportunity to hear conversations that are not normally accessed through one's place in the hierarchy but that may be beneficial to hear. They make boundaries temporarily more permeable, and more visible. What is revealed and experienced within the hour has the potential to deepen understanding of unspoken aspects of healthcare experience, highlight the value of acknowledging true inner experience, and subtly shift staff's relationship to themselves.

Getting it wrong: mistakes, complaints and being human

For a long time we had thought of doing a Round about mistakes. We felt it was important but we were getting large numbers coming to our Rounds and we knew it carried a risk, and would have to be carefully managed. An internet search to plan the Round revealed that the sharing by doctors of stories about their errors was powerful and useful but often took place in uni-disciplinary and smaller settings. But two doctors offered to be on the panel, one talking about attending the coroner's court, the other describing being reported to the GMC, and so I met them both to prepare. The story of the senior clinician being reported to the GMC is the one that stayed with me.

I met him in his office at the back of a large, cluttered, open plan office space. His room was also cluttered, filled with files and books and, though small, it had desks for three consultants: a small, dusty, uncongenial place for the planning of big, important jobs. Like many panel preparation sessions there was little time available and pressure to get a story and a clinician who would both underplay it and then have so much to say: I had become used to the way in which clinicians underestimated their own stories at the same time as needing them to be heard, the need growing stronger as they began to speak.

At the heart of the story was the doctor's huge regret about losing his cool with a family in their hour of need. He had been abrupt and frustrated with them to the point that they did not feel they received the information and the care they needed, and ultimately reported him to the GMC. Once this process is in place an investigation must take place. It is out of the doctors' hands and beyond the remit of the hospital. Along with all the obvious worries many doctors feel abandoned and alone throughout this process. In this case there had been no serious clinical risk but a very poor patient and family experience. The doctor was full of remorse and regrets that he had let them down and extremely relieved that nothing clinically serious had gone wrong. As he told his story it became clear that he had been working under immense pressure at the time of the complaint. The risk he might have being taking by being in work when his personal life was under so much pressure was also apparent.

At the time that the complaint occurred the doctor's clinical lead had become terminally ill, diagnosed tragically and poignantly with the condition he had dedicated his life to treat, just at the point of his retirement. He was like a father to his team, many of whom he had trained, and they were all devastated for him and for themselves as they anticipated the loss of him. As a result the doctor was covering both the clinical lead's work and his own. And at the same time his own father was dying in another hospital and every night when he had finished his work he went and slept on the floor in his father's hospital room. He knew he was pushing his limits but it was just for a week. But it was in this week that the complaint happened.

Medical school narrows the perspective of doctors to focus on the rational and creates a demand for robustness. Bright, competitive, and aspirational medical students rise to this challenge. They have been selected to succeed and so of course they will. And the myth that attending to their own emotional needs is a sign of weakness is unconsciously absorbed and perpetuated. The overwhelming volume of work in NHS hospitals encourages individual staff to collude with its denial of the reality of the finiteness of any one individual's capacity to work, to care, to contribute, and to be productive at work. Into this all too common trap this doctor had strayed at a time of his own need. Now he wanted to tell the story in a Schwartz Round and share the emotions that it had left him with. I wondered why. I found myself, not for the first time, in the position of hearing a very moving personal story during a panel preparation and while the doctor expressed regret and self-criticism, what I was struck by was his integrity and the grief he was going through. The clinical lead had now died and the doctor was preparing to speak at his funeral, which would take place the week after our meeting.

The Round was well attended and many of the doctor's colleagues were in the audience. He told his story factually and clearly, albeit with some hesitations, and the audience were rapt. A young doctor in the audience spoke first to say how much it meant to her to hear a senior and highly respected doctor talk so honestly about this experience. Other members of the audience expressed regret for what he had endured alone, concern for him and the strain he had carried, and also praised him for speaking on the panel. The group discussion was respectful to the experience of the patient and their family, and managed to balance an acknowledgement of the negative experience they had had with a compassionate curiosity about what the experience had been like for the doctor. Once again in a Round I watched the possibility of criticism being dissolved as an authentic panel story was greeted with warm support, recognition of the values that inspired the clinician, which became clear in the storytelling, and concern about the impact of this experience on him.

And then from the back of the room a very senior doctor spoke. He had not seen the strain his colleague was under and the risk he was running but now after listening to the story he could see the effect the experience had had. He was sorry. There was an extraordinary exchange then between him and the panellist doctor within which there was an acknowledgement of how difficult it is for doctors to look after each other, what a difference it might have made for the panel doctor to have felt more overtly supported, how hard it is to tell a senior colleague that he shouldn't be at work, and what a lonely experience being a consultant can be. There was complete stillness in the room during this powerful conversation that would normally have taken place behind closed doors. This stillness remained until the end of the Round, after which many colleagues thanked us for allowing this story to be told. This was acknowledged in the feedback forms and many supportive emails to the doctor in response to his storytelling and honesty.

Afterwards I wondered about how the space within the Round can be used both as a confessional, and as a place where anger can be expressed towards the organisation. And I thought about the value of this if the space is safely contained to allow individual experiences to be safely handed over to the group to share, rather than being carried alone by the storyteller. In this case the organisation is best seen as an entity, an "other" to whom we relate sometimes as if it were a culpable person, a containing parent who has failed us. And don't we need the possibility of this containment, for without it we would be too alone in the murky, hopeful water of healthcare within which the power we have, and the helplessness we simultaneously hold for patients are in constant contact? But we also need the chance to express our disappointment when it feels as if it's failed us.

The Round provided an opportunity for the doctor to express his feelings about what he had had to withstand personally and professionally, both in the events that led to the complaint and then in the difficult process of the complaint investigation. At some level maybe he wanted to speak at the Round in order to both be forgiven for the error, and to express this anger at the intolerable burden he had had to carry. And as if by magic both became possible in this Round that had the unexpected gift of an apology from the "other" and a group acknowledgement and witnessing of the loneliness and isolation of the senior clinician.

Left holding the baby: a tale of strong arms

Some Rounds leave you with a strong visual image which stays with you. One such image is of a tall, strong male nurse sitting for two hours in A&E, holding a baby who had just died while waiting for the baby's family to return. He had promised them he would not let the baby go. Perhaps the image remained because when it came to this man's turn to speak on the panel he stood up (unlike the other panellists) and the contrast between his height, stature, and strength, and the tender way in which he described holding this child, was so poignant and moving that the room was completely gripped, or because of the simple sad fact of a baby dying. Or because this Round had at its heart a case where although nothing could be done to improve the outcome for the child, the care that he and his family received was so exquisitely sensitive. Or perhaps it was that underneath the story was a reality that often emerges in a Schwartz Round—that healthcare staff are often left to do the emotional work that a patient and/or his family are unable to do, for a variety of reasons.

The panel for this Round was a mixture of hospital and community staff. The mother of the baby was a young woman. Prenatal testing had indicated that the baby had a number of problems and that if he survived to birth, he would have poor quality of life and very limited life expectancy. The team made a number of different efforts to help the family to understand this but with no success. The family had some difficulties of their own which made it hard for them to grasp and accept the reality of the situation. The dilemma then became how to keep the baby safe and support the family to look after him when he was born. The baby was delivered and despite needing specialist neonatal care he made it home though he needed ongoing treatment. For the family he simply represented hope, joy, the future, and someone very precious to be cared for. Although they had some difficulties looking after themselves and their home, when it came to the baby everything was different. They dressed him beautifully and cared for him expertly. The young community nurse who made a strong bond with the family visited regularly. She would silently check that everything was safe and in hand, and spend the rest of the time enjoying the baby with his mum, commenting on how lovely the baby's clothes were that day and how well the family was doing. However, at five months old the baby was urgently admitted to A&E, and died there.

All members of the panel described their experience of this work, the sadness, the risk they had had to manage, and the emotional effort put into creatively supporting this family to care for the baby for as long as they had him. The nurse with strong arms was not involved in the work but was in charge in A&E when the baby died. Seeing how shocked the family were he encouraged them to return home to shower and change and promised that he would mind the baby while they were gone. He could also see that his own staff were distressed to see a baby die and he wanted to protect them too. He asked them to keep other patients away from this area of A&E and sat with the baby in his arms for two hours. Protocol dictated that the body should have been moved to the mortuary in this time but he knew that the family would be very distressed by this so he consciously delayed this process until they returned. A member of the audience asked him what the experience of holding the baby for all this time was like—was he sad? He said he had always found holding babies peaceful and that this experience was peaceful too.

This powerful story of wisdom and quiet respectful containment moved people in the audience very much. There was a true sense of pride in the work of their colleagues and in their ability to be flexible and creative. Their appreciation of the meaning of this baby for the family and their sensitivity to this, despite the difficulties the family had and the imminence of their loss, was deeply impressive.

Healthcare workers choose their work because they want to make things better. They hope to heal and they want to repair. But sometimes they can't. It can take a lifetime, or maybe a certain career stage to appreciate this. Sometimes all that can be done is to bear witness. Rounds such as this help with the acceptance of this reality and allow consideration and discussion of the resources that healthcare workers need to draw on in order to be able to bear witness. Through the discussion that followed, the way in which the healthcare workers blended hope, acceptance, active intervention, stepping back, and changing gear to get it right for both the baby and the family became apparent.

The family is the unit in which difficult transitions and their resulting emotional work need to be managed: accepting disability and loss, realising the gap between the hoped for ideal and the eventual outcome, and accepting change. But sometimes this unit is not strong or flexible enough to withstand reality. In this case healthcare workers are often called on to step in to take or share the responsibility required of the family. This happens both explicitly and implicitly and is most often apparent in work with children and the elderly: the joining up of the healthcare system with the family system to allow the unbearable to be borne. This reality has emerged in many different Round stories which are preoccupied with the impact on staff of becoming "in loco parentis". In this case the strong arms of this nurse created a moment of stillness and holding for the baby, the family, and the staff when there was quite simply nothing else that could be done.

Being under public scrutiny: responding without retaliating

In the second year of Rounds we decided to tackle an organisational rather than a clinical experience. The hospital had experienced a difficult summer within which an inspection had been failed and a clinical error with fatal consequences had been widely reported on national television. We held the Round in the autumn. A second inspection had been successfully passed by this time and measures had been put in place to review the background to the clinical error. Four very senior managers agreed to go on the panel for the Round. They had been responsible for receiving the news of failings and addressing the issues it raised. They were asked to talk about the personal and professional impact of this experience and how they managed to implement improvements without retaliating against staff, given the punitive processes that are often unleashed through an inspection process. Due to the sensitivity of the Round they were prepared individually beforehand.

I remember being struck by the immediate willingness of all panellists to participate. In our preparation sessions they showed great honesty and humanity. They were anxious about exposure but prepared to take the risk. I remember feeling anxious about how to keep the Round safe both for individuals and the organisation. Also how to balance compassion for the managers and the experiences they have when mistakes are made (or judged to have been made), with strong feelings about the patients who had been failed in these incidents.[20] In the preparation meetings they told me of their feelings of disappointment and the sadness that the failings had happened. They described shame and self-criticism and the worry that they "had missed something". Despite the improvements made this worry persisted. There was an unspoken sense that people could get hurt within these systems, as well as in the scrutiny process and this didn't just mean patients. The complexity of the multilayered context that has to be managed in healthcare and the anxiety that an important detail could slip out of view was palpable in the storytelling. As was the worry that the wider context was unforgiving, keen to blame, but without enough underpinning support to secure the structure that was under scrutiny.

---

[20] I feel this same tension in writing this tale, as if we cannot have compassion for the managers if patients suffered, or we might deprive the patient by seeking to understand the manager. But I know in truth that we must understand their experience and support it more helpfully otherwise more patients will suffer.

The commitment of each manager to good patient care was clearly evident, as was the difficulty of keeping the system in view when individuals are ultimately so much easier to target. Amidst intolerable emotional pressure the desire to blame provides instant emotional release. The pressure created by resisting the urge for this release and attempting to motivate disillusioned and frightened staff, while hoping that no one above them would turn on them, was palpable. I asked one manager how they coped with all this emotional strain and the unbelievably long hours which they worked. "I go home at night and I drink a lot of wine," she said, "but I won't say that in the Round." "Of course not," I said, "but I guess if you can give an idea of the personal cost of your role that might be useful for people to know about."

I spent an hour preparing this manager and at the end she said, "I feel better for talking," and I was struck again by how much these senior managers carry, how little it is acknowledged by them and by the system, and what a high personal price some of them are paying for doing this job, in this context, right now. They manage tightly run systems, under financial pressure, sometimes with demoralised staff, at a time when the external world (a potent cocktail of society in general, the political system, and of course the media) is unwilling to accept the degree of uncertainty that is part of any human system. When the individual consequences can be so catastrophic, and the burden of hope and idealism which the NHS carries is so heavy, the tendency to be critical is increased. And so the dual reality of healthcare is perpetuated: the need to appear good and to reach targets, and the need to hide the unspeakable possibility of risk and failure. This can create intolerable emotional strain for managers in healthcare that is often denied, not least by them. The systems that train, support, and appraise them draw for the most part on models proven to work in industry and thus can extend this denial of the emotional labour at the heart of the work and restrict access to spaces in which it can be processed.

After the panel preparation sessions all the panellists wrote down their stories and they brought them as a script to the Round. This very rarely happens in Rounds and when it does it is usually done by junior staff, or staff with no experience of public speaking. But these senior managers with wide experience of public speaking brought typed out stories to guide each of their five-minute slots. As if they could forget the experience. As if without a crib sheet, some unacceptable truths might leak out of their story. The risk of being the weak link in the chain, the uncertainty about how much reality the organisation or the outside world could bear, the fear of letting the side down or having the blame trickle back to overwhelm them, created the need for these neatly typed pages they each held onto as they told their stories.

The Round was extremely well attended and afterwards a senior member of staff in the audience said how impressed he was that the organisation was prepared to tackle such a risky issue in this way. I think many people attended out of a feeling of curiosity and then responded to the humanity of the managers. What I remember most though was the senior manager stopping at the end of her story and looking at me and saying to the audience that I had asked her to share with them how she coped. I suddenly felt full of all the anxiety linked to exposure and the responsibility to ensure that dangerous truths can be carried safely. I wondered would she repeat what she had told me in the preparation session. "I go home and drink lots and lots of cups of tea," she said, and brought the house down.

This witty, clever way of telling the truth in public without overtly exposing herself was both impressive and poignant. We all knew she was describing a widely shared coping strategy to deal with the cost of working in an unforgiving system and trying, sometimes under almost impossible pressures, to retain some humanity—for others if not for herself. Almost everyone in the room shared that experience to a greater or lesser extent. And the reality of course is that it may be the health professional who pays the least attention to her own health, and comes to harm in the end. I had already learnt this through the staff who used the therapy service. But in that moment of witty storytelling the split that often exists in healthcare between bad, tough manager and good, kind clinician was impossible to maintain; and the human face of the organisation and the cost of its work was evident in a surprising and honest way.

Letting go: tales of safe passage

A young woman had died of a very painful illness. One of the teams looking after her suggested to me that this would make for a good Round. It had been a very difficult case, caused conflicts between team members, and left some very traumatic memories for staff. In the panel preparation meetings I met with a number of clinicians who winced when they discussed the patient. They were remembering the speedy way the illness had progressed and how this produced the maximum distress for her. All of them spoke about how unlucky she was and how sad they were for her. The pain and relentless loss of function were agonising to watch. The illness meant that all the soft tissue in her body was hardening: lungs, heart, muscle. A number of multidisciplinary teams were supporting her. Many of them felt that the woman was coming to terms with her imminent death but her mother couldn't. She was pushing for very active medical intervention and still hoping for a cure. But constant intervention caused the daughter more pain and distress and was unable to make any impact on the illness. The mother couldn't be persuaded to see this. The case led to many difficult discussions, much thought and reflection, and various efforts to help both the daughter and the mother. Eventually the daughter died one morning on the ward but her mother refused to allow her body to be taken to the mortuary. The chaplain was called. Hospitals have a standard time by which a body is meant to be removed and brought to the mortuary but the chaplain and the nurses knew that this would take as long as it took.

On the Schwartz Round panel the chaplain described his day sitting with the mother and her daughter's body. The thing that I remember most about his story was that the subtle, sensitive work that he did with the mother was achieved paradoxically by being concrete and direct. He did not talk about the meaning of what had happened or her loss or her feelings, nor did he emphasise God or spirituality although his role implied the possibility of that conversation. Instead he opened a space within which he conveyed that he was available but would proceed at her pace and not impose. While having a strong sense of the terrible loss she was confronting he sat with her in silence, breaking it occasionally with some words about the body, about how it had changed and would change now that the daughter was gone. He did not flinch from the reality of a dead body but allowed it to be the focus of attention. He did not convey any sense of urgency though he could see the nurses outside the room checking periodically to try to get a sense of when the bed would be free. He spoke to the mother and he listened to her. Eventually he asked her if she would like to say some prayers that allowed him to begin to put into words the possibility of letting her daughter go, of handing her over to God. He touched the body and pointed out some changes in it. He actively considered how they should relate to it now, and in doing so of course it became undeniable that the woman was gone. By not reacting to her inability to let go and by staying with the mother and not rushing her, he enabled her rigid holding on to begin to soften. Other relatives came and were very distressed. They tried offering the mother comfort but she didn't respond. Eventually she told the chaplain that the porters could bring the body to the mortuary.

The audience were gripped by the way the chaplain told the story, both the awfulness and the simplicity of it, and the way in which he underplayed his contribution. Through bearing witness to an act of desperation without flinching from any aspect of it, he enabled this woman to let go of her daughter's body. By proceeding at the woman's pace he ensured that the sheer impossibility of handing over her only child was not forced on her but slowly became inevitable and shared.

This Round made me think about how modifying a professional role can provide permission for a new relationship to difficulty, when the individual acts in a direction different to the one the role suggests. By being flexible in role and using it in creative ways—a chaplain being concrete and talking about a body and not a spirit, for example, or a surgeon discussing the psychological impact of a surgical procedure—a powerful intervention is made possible because the expected and unexpected are combined. Maybe the surprise created communicates a flexible wisdom that invites trust and a feeling of safety in the relationship. The safety allows the patient or relative to manage fear and to keep moving forward. (Who knows where?) Bringing together the expected and unexpected in one person's behaviour conveys the split realities we all live in. Connecting people in an unexpected way with a traumatic experience that seems unmanageable allows it to begin to be digested. And this flexibility, this drawing together of one's humanity and one's role, is important to the patient, relative, and the clinician. It allows the clinician to draw on reserves of resilience. And these will be needed. Because in the face of the impossible realities of birth and death, which we mostly (and of necessity) keep out of view in "ordinary" life, healthcare workers are providing safe passage to strangers, even in the direst of circumstances, every day.

My family and other organisations that I have belonged to:
tales of family at home and work

One Christmas, a very senior nurse consultant was retiring. Over twenty-five years in the hospital she had made an enormous contribution both as an innovative clinician and leader but also as a source of organisational intelligence and wisdom, often drawn on to tackle organisational difficulties and challenges. Schwartz Rounds had been running for five years and among other things it was clear that they had become a community meeting and as such they could be used to mark the contribution that this nurse had made to the hospital community. However, a Round is not a leaving party and so we decided to develop a Round along a theme of "becoming a consultant" and to include other clinicians. The panel ultimately comprised three female nurse consultants and one male medical consultant, all of whom had spent a significant proportion of their careers at the hospital. It is the panel preparation that I remember most.

The two other nurse consultants, like the nurse who was leaving, had risen through the ranks to become clinical leads in their specialties—a role traditionally taken by doctors. Looking back, what had initially felt incidental in the choices of how to approach the event (we want to celebrate the retiring nurse, who else can we have on the panel?; we have diverse stories, why don't we create a focus around becoming a consultant?, etc.) seemed to have a design, as stories emerged which unexpectedly reflected history: both family history and the history of the hospital. The process by which stories push through to be heard became worth considering in this Round. Do we choose them or did they choose us? Something deeper than a story of three women and a man, of four clinicians, seemed to be at work in this Round.

During the course of the panel preparation I was left with a strong sense of the three nurses as pioneers, extending the role of the nurse consultant, and the power and influence of female clinicians in a traditional male, medical hierarchy. Through the storytelling the way in which the culture had provided opportunities for these women to be creative and innovative became apparent to all of us, as well as how skilled they had been in capitalising on these opportunities. In some ways it also seemed, as the stories deepened, that the panellists developed a new appreciation for the freedom they been allowed to draw on, and how they had maximised this in order to innovate and to integrate nursing values and ideals into the services they had designed. As this theme emerged I suddenly glimpsed the freedom that, looking back, I had also had as a psychologist to develop the psychology service within the hospital at that time. This panel preparation session helped us all to understand the interaction between our hopes for our profession and careers, and the organisation in which we found ourselves.

I asked all the women to think of a pivotal moment in their career when they had thought, "Yes, this is it, this is what I am meant to be doing," and also to bring to mind who in their family, alive or dead, would have been unsurprised to see them achieve what they had in their career. These questions prompted the following memories.

One of the nurses described being at a meeting in Westminster about end of life care in which difficult, contentious issues were being discussed at a time of much national anxiety about the direction of end of life policy. She felt the need to disagree with a point that was being made, in a way that would bring the reality of the dying patient's experience into the room, and she spoke clearly and emphatically, ensuring that the strong voice of a clinician could advocate for the patient. At the moment when she finished speaking she heard Big Ben strike. She suddenly remembered her grandmother who had attended university in Wales in the 1900s and thought how proud she would be to see her here at the heart of the Department of Health arguing for the values that informed all of her clinical practice and drawing on a family history of innovation and challenge.

The other nurse consultant described how unafraid she was of being seen as "bolshie" or contentious, unafraid to challenge or be unpopular and have people disagree with her, and how she had never felt the need to be a pleaser in the development of her service. The memory of the first nurse had prompted her to think of her own grandparents, and specifically her great-grandfather, a nonconformist liberal who had been involved in the foundation of the *Manchester Guardian*, and how he would have been pleased to see her challenge the medical establishment and its traditional roles and expectations of female clinicians. This then prompted the first nurse to remember her own great-grandfather who had been a strong presence in the development of the nonconformist Church in Wales.

Neither knew of each other's back story; the panel preparation created this new connection between them in this unexpected link to the past and appreciation of the memories that now surfaced with a sudden recognition of their influence on the present. The third nurse consultant spoke of a weekend working with her father, a senior manager in a shipping firm during a strike when a number of ships had been dangerously abandoned in the port. She was a teenage girl at the time and described helping him to tether large ships in the port. It seemed that he expected nothing less. The can-do and practical attitude that he had inspired in her had been carried into the setting up of her service.

It became clear that all three women were assertive problem solvers and doers, with strong role models, and had worked with male consultants who had both supported and challenged them and vice versa. Within these relationships, differences had become creative and synergistic. This synergistic space in which there was conflict, challenge, argument, respect, black humour, and bad language (the push and pull and role reversals of difference—male versus female, nurse versus doctor, carer versus critic), was the space within which these clinicians were able to keep something human—the patient, their values, their energy—at the heart of the services they designed and close to the other clinicians they inspired.

All of them seemed to have managed to stay in touch with the essence of clinical work, its pleasures and challenges, while rising to very senior levels of management. They could connect the personal to the political reality of organisational life. They had managed to hustle effectively within its marketplace where resources are fought for, priorities argued out, target setting success and failure begins and ends careers, and where the silent voices of vulnerable patients can so easily be drowned out. Perhaps the ability to keep these voices in mind in the noisy marketplace of modern healthcare is a part of the flexibility with which successful clinical leaders move positions—from male to female, carer to competitor, soother to aggressor, pacifier to catalyst—within *themselves*, in order to be creative in clinical work and service delivery.

They were joined on the panel by a male consultant who like them had trained at the hospital. He is the consultant from the first of these tales, whose father had founded the transplant service in which he worked and given him his love for the work. And so, quite unexpectedly, the panel stories became stories of family and not just family memories, but the family within the hospital in which all four clinicians had matured, created their own teams, and done good for countless families. The Round itself provided an opportunity for audience members to acknowledge how these clinicians had inspired them in their careers, and the contribution they had made to the life of the organisation.

As they told their stories in the Round, three things suddenly struck me. First, the hospital had recently gone through a merger. This experience of a contrasting culture seemed to be making the positive aspects of the original hospital's culture easier to see and reflect on and this became apparent in each story. I realised how easy it is to become trapped in the narrative of negativity that pervades NHS culture. A sudden experience of contrast, and perhaps a wave of nostalgia, connected each story to positive aspects of the experience of the original culture. Second, I suddenly (and belatedly!) remembered that the hospital had been the first in the country to train women doctors and wondered if this foundation continued to create a space within which strong female clinicians can craft services with authority. The complex culture of healthcare within which overt hierarchies contain hidden possibilities, with permission to use them, perhaps unconsciously available because of past history, was apparent in the stories. And finally, I reflected how, despite all the negative aspects of healthcare culture, which are so evident, and so regularly discussed in wider societal culture, this context had allowed four creative and innovative clinicians to bring together different aspects of themselves, their history, and their organisation, in a way that allowed them to flourish. They had created a sense of family within each of their teams, which honoured and reflected the histories they came from. And now in the room as the stories were being told, a sense of family within the organisation was palpable. The move from accident to design in the emergence of these themes suggested to me that something unconscious may have been at work in a Round that seemed ultimately to be about allowing stories of history, flexibility, and creativity to be told at a time of change, and the end of an era. I had long wondered about the stories that needed to be told finding their way into Rounds—which reveal the connection between the personal and the professional, but now I began to wonder about the way in which they could also reveal connections between the personal and the political …

For they have so many layers, these stories, and often reveal the unconscious reciprocity between our present, and our past, our selves, and the careers we choose. The push and pull, between our work and our lives, our public and private selves. And once the choices are made, the resulting ways in which our work, and this tussle, continue to form us. Now the use of this space for stories of the organisation to emerge, stories of its history and culture and ancestors, and for voices from the past to continue to push through to be heard, began to suggest itself.

And maybe this undertow of suggestion is the cumulative impact of the repetitive, tidal process of preparing and crafting stories for the simple purpose of being spoken and of being heard in public, with no other end in mind, which we have embarked upon. It allows the messy complexity of individual and organisational life in healthcare to take a discernible form, to be temporarily coherent in a structured and regular way, to have a beginning, a middle, and an end, like all the best stories do. Though in truth we know that we are just muddling our way through the part where the final shape is unclear and where beginnings, middles, and ends (ours, our patients', our organisations') are tangled up together blindly in the course of a simple day at work.

PART **V**

Untold stories and unfinished business

Some closing thoughts on working in healthcare

Getting started, keeping going, getting started again—in art and in life, it seems to me this is the essential rhythm not only of achievement but of survival, the ground of convinced action, the basis of self-esteem and the guarantee of credibility in your lives, credibility to yourselves as well as to others.

Seamus Heaney, Finders Keepers, 2002

Untold stories and unfinished business

Sixteen years of being a psychologist in a hospital, six years of running Rounds. So many secrets. So many stories. All those invitations to learn, to see, to witness, to listen and understand. Healthcare work is so rich and meaningful. Healthcare organisations are so troubled, yet so full of people who want to care, to help, to learn and make a difference. The wider context of public sector organisations is so challenged. The problems we face now have no easy solutions. The need to think, feel, *and* act in a connected way so imperative.

Providing spaces in which these connections can be made is so important. Listening neutrally. Allowing form to emerge without judgement. Offering solace and comfort, and clarity. Helping people craft their story for a public telling but to no other end has proved to be a powerful experience for them and for the listeners. Keeping an eye on context. Trying to move in the opposite direction to busyness in order to create options. Linking the incompatibles. Finding a position in which the bridge between inner, private experience and outer, publicly sanctioned stories can be made visible, so useful.

The work done in healthcare is powerful, the chances to cure increasing all the time. The opportunity to be with patients and their families at their time of greatest need, their moments of rawness and vulnerability, is so rewarding and satisfying. Everyone who has lost someone or been through a serious illness or trauma is infinitely grateful to healthcare staff. In the middle of a totally unwanted experience they suddenly see the goodness in humanity, a hundred acts of thoughtfulness, kindness, and care, and impressive, sophisticated clinical skills. Often they find they are having the worst experience of their life at a time they see the best in people. They never forget but the lucky ones are glad to leave this world behind, to leave the hospital and get back to the real world.

Healthcare staff don't get to leave. They have to stay. They have to live in both worlds at the same time. But they know how lucky they are to be doing meaningful work. They know the power that they have at their fingertips. They have a secret. They can keep us alive. They can give us safe passage when we are dying. We need them. They don't have ordinary jobs, they work right on the edge of mystery and understanding.

The invisible cost to them of this powerful secret can take its toll, especially if their organisation struggles to support them in digesting the emotional complexity of their work. Undigested experiences create toxins that seep into the membranes of healthcare organisations and their staff, blocking thinking, disrupting creativity, paving the way for blindness and dysfunction. Psychology can create space, craft story, support the connection to emotion, provide solace, and open up opportunities to witness the reality of individual and organisational life in healthcare. It can provide moments of coherence to enable staff to nurture and sustain themselves so that they can continue to work and to love. That is, to maintain a public and a private life, in an integrated way. To work and to love in the outer world of the organisation and also in their inner world, which can become so cluttered by the impossible dance of organisational life.

Courage and a half-begun story

On a trip home to Dublin I visited some family friends. Their father is a retired anaesthetist and asked me about my work. I told him about a recent Round that we had done called "A patient I will never forget". "Yes," he said, "we all have them." He told me about an eight-year-old girl from years ago about to have risky, essential surgery, and frightened. On the operating table she raised her arm when he held her hand for the injection needle, looked deep into his eyes and said: "Don't." He comforted her and then anaesthetised her.

"Don't" was her last word: she died on the operating table. He still thinks of her. We were sitting in the conservatory in his house looking out on a beautiful Dublin spring garden, when he told me this story. Quickly, simply, no fuss. A wise, kind man I have known all my life. I've listened to and loved so many of his stories and the warm way he tells them since I was little. He has four children of his own, my friends, who I imagine he came home to on that night of the little girl's death. Brave people these clinicians are. Tough stories they carry with them, that have to be put to bed, so families can be taken care of, and other children can sleep at night.

Wheels within wheels, in the hospital world of life, death, and survival. Who knows who will get the happy ending or who will have to leave before their story seems to be over? What do we do with the broken bits, the half-told stories that are left behind and that get carried in our bodies and our minds? The uncertainty, and the unfinished business? How do we make sure that we can keep living and caring for those who need us while allowing the spirit of those who had to leave to surge right through us, to keep us on the right side of the line, where courage, hope, and perseverance remain possible, until we too have to go?

It's the incompleteness of the work that leaves us craving coherent spaces. It's the unavoidably fragmented nature of organisational life right now, that needs to be named and stared down, just to keep us on our toes, to remind us that there is no other perfect place. We are only passing through, flicking away the flotsam and the jetsam, looking for our jewels, unsure where the story ends, happy to be here, keen to be creative in our work, unable to build an organisation that can contain us. It's the stories that will hold us when nothing else can. The memory of those hours, when we could hear a tale that had a beginning, a middle, and an end. That had a form that could sustain us. Ever since we were little the stories have kept the darkness at bay. That and each other will get us through.

REFERENCES

Armstrong, D., & Rustin, M. (Eds.) (2015). Introduction: Revisiting the paradigm. In: *Social Defences Against Anxiety: Explorations in a Paradigm*. London: Karnac.

Berwick, D. (2013). *A Promise to Learn, a Commitment to Act: the Berwick Review into Patient Safety*. London: Department of Health.

Bettelheim, B. (1976). *The Uses of Enchantment*. New York: Vintage, 2010.

Bruner, J. (1986). *Actual Minds, Possible Worlds*. Boston, MA: Beacon Press.

Carey, M., & Russell, S. (2013). Outsider witness practices: some answers to commonly asked questions. *International Journal of Narrative Therapy and Community Work, 1*. Adelaide, Australia: Department for Child Protection.

Firth-Cozens, J., & Cornwell, J. (2009). *Enabling Compassionate Care in Acute Hospital Settings*. London: The King's Fund.

Francis, R. (2013). *Report of the Mid Staffordshire NHS Foundation Trust Public Inquiry*. London: House of Commons. ISBN 9780102981476.

Fredman, G., & Reder, P. (1996). The relationship to help: Interacting beliefs about the treatment process. *Clinical Child Psychology and Psychiatry, 1*: 457–467.

Freedman, J., & Coombs, G. (1996). *The Social Construction of Preferred Realities*. New York: W. W. Norton.

Goodrich, J., & Cornwell, J. (2008). *Seeing the Person in the Patient*. London: The King's Fund.

Goodrich, J., & Levenson, R. (2011). Supporting hospital staff to provide compassionate care: Do Schwartz Center rounds work in English hospitals? *Journal of the Royal Society of Medicine*, 105: 117–122.

Heaney, S. (1995). The Nobel Lecture on the acceptance of the Nobel Prize for Literature, Oslo.

Heaney, S. (2002). *Finders Keepers*. London: Faber & Faber.

Menzies, I. (1960). A case study in the functioning of social systems against anxiety: a report on the study of the nursing service in a general hospital. *Human Relations*, 13(2): 95–121.

Menzies Lyth, I. (1988). *Containing Anxiety in Institutions: Selected Essays*. London: Free Association.

Obholzer, A. (1994). Managing social anxieties in public sector organisations. In: A. Obholzer & V. Z. Roberts (Eds.), *The Unconscious at Work*. London: Routledge.

Pearce, W. B. (1976). The co-ordinated management of meaning: a rules based theory of interpersonal communication. In: G. R. Miller (Ed.), *Explorations in Interpersonal Communication* (pp. 17–36). Newbury Park, CA: Sage.

Schwartz, K. B. (1995). A patient's story. *The Boston Globe Magazine*, 16 July. Available from http://www.theschwartzcenter

White, M. (2014). Working with people who are suffering from the consequences of multiple trauma: A narrative perspective. *International Journal of Narrative Therapy and Community Work*, 1: 45–76.

Williams, S., Michie, S., & Pattani, S. (1998). Improving the Health of the NHS Workforce: Report of the Partnership on the Health of the NHS Workforce. London: Nuffield Trust.

Wren, B. (2012). Schwartz Rounds: Creating new spaces and having new conversations in healthcare. [Paper presented at OPUS International Conference, London.]

Wren, B. (2013). Setting Up and Running Schwartz Center Rounds *A Practical Handbook*. London: Point of Care Foundation.

Wren, B. (2014). Schwartz rounds: An intervention with potential to simultaneously improve staff experience and organisational culture. *Clinical Psychology Forum*, 263: 22–25.

Wren, B. (2015). Developing training for Schwartz Round facilitators and clinical leads: harnessing hope and developing creativity in tough organizational contexts. [Paper presented at OPUS International Conference, London.]

Yeats, W. B. (1919). The second coming. *The Dial*.

Yeats, W. B. (1928). Among school children. In: R. J. Finneran (Ed.), *The Poems of W. B. Yeats: A New Edition*. London: Macmillan, 1933.

INDEX